CAESAREAN BIRTH

your questions answered

Debbie Chippington Derrick

Gina Lowdon

Fiona Barlow

 The National Childbirth Trust

Published 2004 by The National Childbirth Trust
Alexandra House, Oldham Terrace, London W3 6NH

© National Childbirth Trust 2004

ISBN 0-9543018-3-8

The National Childbirth Trust

The National Childbirth Trust wants all parents to have an experience of pregnancy, birth and early parenthood that enriches their lives and gives them confidence in being a parent.

To find out where your nearest National Childbirth Trust group is, ring the NCT enquiry line on 0870 444 8707.

www.nctpregnancyandbabycare.com

You are welcome to use NCT services whether you are a member or not. However, more members mean more resources to help us continue our work for parents. To join the NCT with a credit or debit card, please ring 0870 990 8040.
We welcome donations to support our charity.
For a full list of publications, write to

NCT Sales
239 Shawbridge Street
Glasgow G43 1QN
or contact 0870 112 1120
www.nctms.co.uk

Acknowledgements

The NCT and the authors would like to thank all the women who shared their experiences of caesarean birth with us.

Editorial	Alison Turnbull, Fit to Print
Page design	Jane Evans Design
Cover photograph and design	Mel Colton, Chemistry Group
Review team	Mary Newburn
	Cynthia Clarkson
	Roz Collins
Panel representatives	Julie Jones (breastfeeding counsellor)
	Cynthia Masters-Waage (antenatal teacher)
	Helen Bates (antenatal teacher)
	Sharon Tong (postnatal leader)
Anaesthetics review	Dr Geraldine O'Sullivan, President.
	Obstetric Anaesthetists' Association

Contents

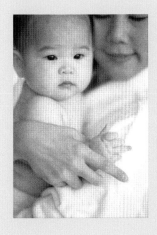

Contents *continued*

Foreword

The NCT has done such a lot to inform families about maternity care and to encourage midwives and obstetricians to think about how their care affects women and babies. This booklet was successful in its first edition and is even more necessary now. In 1996, when it was first published, one in seven babies was born by caesarean section.

Now, about one in five mothers in the UK has a caesarean – around 150,000 of the 669,000 giving birth each year. This booklet will let women and their families know:

- why a caesarean may be advised

- what choices and decisions they can make

- what to expect during and after the operation.

This booklet includes answers to all kinds of frequently asked questions based on up-to-date evidence and a sensitivity to women's needs and feelings. It also provides lots of practical tips and quotes from parents' experiences. The NCT also publishes information sheets on *Straightforward birth*, *Breech baby* and *Vaginal birth after a caesarean*, which include information about what can be done to reduce the need for a caesarean.

This booklet complements the newly published evidence-based guideline on Caesarean Section by the National Institute for Clinical Effectiveness (NICE)[1] which should be used by health professionals in England and Wales, and will also be referred to in Scotland and Northern Ireland.

Susan Bewley
Consultant Obstetrician
Guy's & St Thomas' Hospital NHS Trust

Introduction

Many books have been written about pregnancy and childbirth, but it is not easy to find clear and detailed information about caesarean birth and what happens afterwards. Each of the authors has had at least one baby by caesarean. When we were pregnant, and afterwards, we found that it was difficult to find reliable answers to our questions.

It is still surprisingly difficult to find good information – even with access to the Internet parents are often not able to find out what they want to know.

In this second edition of *Caesarean Birth: your questions answered* we have brought together personal experiences and the latest available research, including that from the guideline published in April 2004 by the National Institute of Clinical Excellence.[1] One of us was a member of the guideline development group.

In this booklet we aim to:

- answer common questions about caesarean birth
- provide further information about this way of giving birth
- point you to the wide range of people and organisations who can support you – professionally, emotionally and practically
- help parents who leave hospital feeling they do not fully understand their caesarean experience.

Whichever way your baby is born, most of the joys and challenges of early parenthood are similar for all parents.

Debbie Chippington Derrick

Gina Lowdon

Fiona Barlow

June 2004

About caesareans

What is a caesarean?

A caesarean section is an operation in which the baby is born through a cut in the woman's abdomen.

An 'elective' caesarean is planned before the woman goes into labour, sometimes even early in pregnancy.

An 'emergency' caesarean is not planned before labour. The decision is taken any time from 10 minutes to a few hours before the operation, depending on how urgently an intervention is needed. In almost two-thirds of UK caesareans the decision to have a caesarean is taken during labour.[2]

Why have a caesarean?

Clear evidence

In some cases, there is clear evidence that a caesarean is needed to save life or reduce the risks for mother or baby. A caesarean is clearly indicated in the case of:

- cord prolapse
- some malpositions of the baby
- some medical conditions of the baby
- placenta praevia
- severe placental abruption
- severe pre-eclampsia
- severely impaired fetal growth
- suspected uterine rupture.

"The advantages were huge apart from not being able to drive. I could plan for the birth and carried on working until the last day, was able to breastfeed OK and returned to work when she was three months old."

"Having attended antenatal classes, I was convinced of the 'rightness' of a natural birth. But having given it my best shot, I do not feel a failure for not producing my child unaided. On the contrary, I am proud of myself and my husband."

What do these medical terms mean?

Cord prolapse: When the umbilical cord comes down into the vagina in front of the baby.

Malposition of the baby: Towards the end of pregnancy, babies usually settle in the uterus with their head down, facing their mother's back. Some babies settle in ways that can make birth more complicated. These include:

- transverse or oblique lie, when the baby lies horizontally or diagonally in the uterus. It may be possible to turn the baby, especially if the waters have not broken

- brow first, which puts a larger diameter of the baby's head into the pelvis. Good contractions may alter the position of the baby's head during labour and make vaginal birth possible

- face first, with the baby's chin towards the mother's spine

- 'star-gazing' breech, when the baby is in the breech position with the neck extended.

Medical conditions: Some medical conditions of the baby may be incompatible with vaginal birth for some cases of the following:

- heart conditions

- hydrocephalus (head enlarged by 'water on the brain')

- some tumours.

Placenta praevia: The placenta lies across, or less than two centimetres from the neck of the uterus, towards the end of pregnancy or when labour starts.

"My baby was lying completely transverse with the cord prolapsed. It was obvious that it would have to be a caesarean. The midwife had to keep her hand on the cord (inside me) until the operation was performed."

"I didn't feel at all cheated at having a caesarean – I was so pleased to have a live baby, and was shocked that I had come so close to losing him."

2

Severe placental abruption: The placenta comes away from the wall of the uterus. In this rare but serious situation, a caesarean will need to be carried out promptly to save the baby's life.

Severe pre-eclampsia: This is a serious medical condition of pregnancy. If pre-eclampsia goes unchecked, the woman may progress to eclampsia and start having fits. This condition is life-threatening and treatment will include delivering the baby. Symptoms of pre-eclampsia include:

- high blood pressure
- swelling caused by water retention (oedema) often noticed first in the legs and arms
- a high level of protein in the urine
- visual disturbances, for example, flashing lights, sensitivity to light, blurred vision
- severe pain in the upper abdomen, under the ribs, like bad heartburn, which may move up to the shoulders.

In less severe cases of pre-eclampsia, induced vaginal delivery is usually an option.

Severely impaired fetal growth: The baby is not getting enough food and oxygen from the placenta and cannot withstand labour. This is difficult to diagnose accurately.

Suspected uterine rupture: The uterus tears, including cases when a uterine scar from previous surgery (caesarean or otherwise) separates. A scar can sometimes begin to come apart without causing problems and without having any effects on labour or delivery. See *Can I have my next baby normally?* on page 71.

IUGR: Intrauterine growth retardation – a term used for impaired fetal growth

"The scar had separated and torn either side, and the baby was in my abdomen, from where they delivered him. The worst part of the whole experience was not believing it when they said he was fine, which he was."

3

Divided opinion

Often the evidence that a caesarean is the best way for a baby to be born is less clear. In some cases, obstetricians have differing opinions on the need for a caesarean. These opinions are not always based on the available medical evidence and different obstetricians may read the same evidence in different ways.

Parents may have different priorities when making decisions. Sometimes the choice about the mode of birth is left to parents. If you feel you do not have enough information on which to base an informed decision, you can seek further information (see *Further support and information,* pages 75-79) and you have a right to be referred for a second opinion.

Cases when professional opinion is divided include:

- breech presentation
- cephalopelvic disproportion
- fibroids
- mother's disability
- existing medical conditions
- failure to progress
- fetal distress
- genital herpes
- HIV
- large baby
- multiple birth
- poor obstetric history
- pre-term labour

"Although he asked us to make the decision, we had little information to base the decision on. What were the risks of either course of action? We didn't ask – but I wish I had. We left the hospital with many questions."

- previous caesarean
- psychological reasons
- previous traumatic birth experience
- unstable lie.

What do these medical terms mean?

Breech presentation: When the baby continues to lie bottom down instead of turning head down. A recent randomised controlled trial showed that planned caesarean birth reduces the number of deaths and the need for resuscitation in full-term breech babies.[3,4] However, there is continuing debate about whether vaginal breech birth is more risky than a caesarean birth for all breech babies, and if so, how much more risky. Some experts have found weaknesses in the way the trial was designed.[5] Some NHS maternity services and independent midwives continue to provide support for vaginal birth for breech babies.

Cephalopelvic disproportion (CPD): When it is thought that the baby's head will not fit through the woman's pelvis. Extreme cases are now rare in the UK as illnesses such as rickets are now very unusual.

CPD is extremely difficult to diagnose. During labour, the baby's head moulds to fit through the pelvis and the pelvis changes size as ligaments stretch. Lying on your back or sitting can compromise the size of the pelvic diameter.[6]

Fibroids: Benign growths of tissue on the wall of the uterus. In some cases, these are large or positioned awkwardly and may affect the position of the baby or prevent a vaginal delivery.

Full-term: sometimes abbreviated to 'term', means that the pregnancy has lasted to at least 37 weeks, or more

ECV: External cephalic version – moving the baby to a head down position by gently turning it from the outside.

ECV can be used to turn as many as half of all full-term breech babies into a head down position so that a caesarean for breech presentation is no longer an issue.

"I would have much preferred a vaginal birth, but could not find anyone with the confidence or experience of delivering breech babies."

5

Disability: Sometimes a disability may make a caesarean necessary. However, obstetricians may recommend a caesarean due to lack of experience. For example, they may assume that a woman who uses a wheelchair must have a caesarean.

Existing medical conditions: Some women with heart disease or diabetes may be advised to have a caesarean.

Failure to progress: When the cervix opens very slowly, and progress does not match clinical expectations. A slow or long labour does not usually put the baby at risk.

Fetal distress: When the baby is thought not to be getting enough oxygen. Research has shown that continuous electronic fetal monitoring (CEFM) for all women has increased the number of babies thought to be in distress.

Using CEFM for all women has raised the rate of caesarean births, but has not improved health outcomes for babies. When fetal distress is suspected, fetal blood sampling reduces unnecessary caesareans.[7,8]

Genital herpes: A skin disease that causes open sores on the genitals from time to time. A caesarean is recommended for all women with first-episode genital herpes lesions at the time of birth or in the last three months of pregnancy.[9] However, a caesarean is not recommended for recurrent genital herpes at the time of delivery, although some obstetricians still advise all women with genital herpes to have a caesarean.

Human immunodeficiency virus (HIV): The virus that may develop into AIDS. Elective caesarean section reduces the transmission of the virus from mother to baby independently of the mother's viral load and whether she is receiving anti-retroviral treatment.[10]

"I wasn't happy about the idea of a caesarean at first. But after researching my situation on the internet, I decided it was best for me and my baby."

Large baby: Large babies born to diabetic mothers have better outcomes if born by elective caesarean. Surgery can protect against shoulder dystocia, (problems in delivering the baby's shoulders after the head is born). However, it is very difficult to predict the size of the unborn baby either by palpation (feeling the abdomen) or ultrasound.

Multiple birth: Some obstetricians recommend a caesarean for all multiple births. Others recommend vaginal delivery of twins if there are no complications and depending on the position of the babies in the uterus – even triplets have been delivered vaginally.

Poor obstetric history or 'precious baby': These terms are sometimes used when a woman has had many miscarriages or a stillbirth, is over 40 years or has had fertility treatment.

Pre-term labour: Labour that starts before the 37th week of pregnancy. Some premature babies may be less able to withstand labour.

Previous caesarean: Women who have had two or more previous caesareans may be advised to have another planned operation, although there seems to be no clear evidence of improved outcomes compared with the outcomes for a vaginal birth.[11,12]

Psychological reasons: Some women have a fear of childbirth (sometimes known as tokophobia). These women can sometimes be helped to view labour more positively through counselling. If not, a psychological assessment can provide a valid medical reason for caesarean delivery.

Previous traumatic birth experience: Either a caesarean or vaginal birth that caused emotional or physical problems.

"... so my 10lb baby was not even 8lbs when they delivered him."

"Other people's reactions were also spectacular. On being told that Adam was very premature, someone actually said to me, 'it must have been a really easy birth then?'!!!! I couldn't believe anyone could be so insensitive."

Unstable lie: When the baby's position in the uterus keeps changing, increasing the risk of cord prolapse.

How safe is a caesarean?

Safety is about weighing up alternative risks and benefits. For each individual, the question to answer is: 'Is there reason to believe that in my case a vaginal birth would carry more risk than a caesarean section?'

Mother's safety

In some cases, a caesarean is the safest way for a baby to be born. However, a caesarean section is major abdominal surgery. Risks to a woman's health include the following:

- anaesthetic complications

- blood clots in the circulation (deep vein thrombosis or thrombo-embolism). Women undergoing surgery should be given drugs and other treatments, such as support stockings, to reduce this risk

- damage to the bladder or bowel during the operation

- endometritis (inflammation of the lining of the uterus)

- future obstetric complications, including reduced fertility, a small increase in stillbirth and the need for emergency hysterectomy

- haemorrhage (severe bleeding)

- infections of the abdominal wound. Infections have been reduced by the use of antibiotics given during surgery, but do still occur

- psychological effects, including depression and post-traumatic stress disorder

- septicaemia (blood poisoning).

Although complications can be life-threatening, the risk of a woman dying after a caesarean is very small, but is greater than for a vaginal delivery.[13] However, it is not known how many maternal deaths result from existing conditions and how many from complications of surgery.

Baby's safety

Caesarean operations undoubtedly save some babies' lives or reduce damage to their health. But there are still risks.

The major risk for the baby is respiratory distress (breathing difficulties), which may be caused by the baby being premature. Babies born by caesarean without their mother having been in labour are at a higher risk of respiratory distress than babies born vaginally at the same gestational age.[14,15,16]

Sometimes it is difficult to deliver a baby by caesarean, and occasionally, the baby may be bruised or cut during the operation. This may also happen if the baby is delivered vaginally using forceps or ventouse.

Could my baby die?

Sadly, a caesarean section does not guarantee a live baby. Despite improvements in obstetric and neonatal care, some babies still die. If your baby dies, you will need time to come to terms with what has happened.

It is important that you get support and information from the professionals who are caring for you, so

"Crossing the front doorstep without our baby Kate was just awful. The phone was an absolute lifeline. The people who were prepared to listen – my midwife, my NCT antenatal group, my SANDS befriender, our family and friends – were all fantastic. They helped me pick up the confidence to try again, and supported me through my oh-so-frightening second pregnancy. And my health visitor, bless her, even put Kate's birthday in her diary and sent me flowers a year later."

that you feel able to decide what happens to you and your baby.

It will be important to do what feels right for you, and in your own time. Many bereaved parents, but not all, have found it helpful to:

- spend private, quiet time with their baby
- name their baby
- bathe and dress their baby, or have their midwife do so
- take photos
- keep mementoes such as a lock of hair or a footprint
- hold a religious or secular ceremony
- have their baby at home with them for a while.

Most hospitals have special bereavement rooms that will also accommodate your partner, but you may be anxious to leave hospital early to grieve in private at home. After a caesarean this will not always be possible. It is likely that you will have some physical pain from the surgery and also when your breasts fill with milk.

It may be helpful to talk to the professionals who are caring for you, who will want to help, but may not understand your needs.

The Stillbirth and Neonatal Death Society (SANDS) offers support to parents after the loss of a baby, including a 24-hour helpline. You'll find their details on page 79.

About your options

Can I choose a caesarean?

Although you do not have a right to a caesarean most obstetricians do respect personal preferences.

Your request will be taken more seriously if you can be clear about your reasons for preferring caesarean birth and if you can show that you are making an 'informed decision' – that you have a good understanding of the risks involved and the realities of the recovery.

The most common reason for wanting a caesarean is to avoid a repeat of a previous traumatic birth experience. If this is your first baby, you may have a fear of childbirth or may have been frightened by what you have heard from others.

The NICE caesarean guideline now encourages obstetricians to refer women requesting a caesarean for counselling.[1] Addressing fears supportively can make a real difference. If a woman can be helped to view labour more positively she may feel more comfortable to give it a try, but if not then a caesarean can be scheduled on the basis of psychological need.

Some women have come to understand that in their particular case it would be safer for their baby to be born by caesarean. If there are clear indications that this is indeed the case, it is unlikely that an obstetrician would refuse a request for a caesarean.

In most cases, if both mother and baby are healthy and there are no psychological reasons, then it is safer and more beneficial for the baby to be born vaginally.

Women who have already had at least one caesarean or who have had a previous difficult vaginal delivery will find any request for a caesarean delivery is accepted more readily.

Other reasons women want to have a caesarean delivery include:

- concern about damage to the perineum – the delicate area between the vagina and the anus – especially if there has been previous trauma

- having a disability, illness, or long-term condition, such as back pain

- previous sexual abuse.

Discuss any concerns you have with your consultant or midwife, or contact a support organisation for more information (see *Who can help?* page 58).

If you want a caesarean delivery you have the right to ask for one. Consultant obstetricians also have the right to say no if they feel that an operation cannot be justified in terms of the possible and likely benefits outweighing the possible and likely harms.

Consultants are sometimes reluctant to consent to caesarean delivery without a clear medical indication. The NICE caesarean guideline states that 'maternal request is not on its own a reason for caesarean section' and encourages obstetricians to explore, discuss and record women's views, ensuring that they understand the benefits and risks of a caesarean compared with vaginal birth.[1] You have the right to seek a second opinion within the NHS or NHS Scotland if you want to discuss your wishes with another obstetrician.

If you want a caesarean delivery and do not have the support of an NHS obstetrician you may wish to make enquiries about private maternity care.

"An elective caesarean was booked for my due date. I felt strange about knowing when my baby would be born. I was overjoyed when, two days before, my waters broke – I would get to feel what labour pain felt like."

Can I choose my anaesthetic?

Three kinds of anaesthetic are usually available for a caesarean. Two forms of regional anaesthetic, spinal block and epidural, numb the lower part of your body so that you can stay awake while your baby is born. General anaesthetic sends you to sleep so that you are not aware of what is happening. Regional anaesthetic is generally preferred because it is safer for mother and baby. If you would like more information about your choices, whether or not a caesarean is booked, you can ask for an appointment with an anaesthetist.

Here we describe each of the three main forms of anaesthetic. Their advantages and disadvantages are compared on pages 14-15.

Spinal block

A spinal block is a single injection of anaesthetic fluid into the spinal column. It makes you numb from your ribcage down, but lets you stay awake and aware of noises and sensations.

You will be asked either to curl over your bump (if you are sitting) or curve around your bump (if you are lying on your side) while the anaesthetist gives a single injection into the fluid in your spinal column. Your birth partner should be able to stay with you while this takes place.

The anaesthetist will check the pain relief in your abdomen and thighs with a cold spray, ice or a light touch. If you can feel pain, say so. A spinal block cannot be topped up like an epidural, although new techniques can now combine a spinal with an epidural. In rare cases when pain relief is not complete you can usually be given a general anaesthetic.

"I have had four elective caesareans, each with spinal anaesthesia. I have thoroughly enjoyed each 'op', found them painless and any pain after easily remedied by painkillers. I think it's a wonderful way to have a baby; the scar is unnoticeable. I have come home after three nights in hospital each of the last times."

13

Anaesthetics compared

	Spinal
Method	Anaesthetic given by a single injection into your spinal column
Timing and top-ups	Cannot be topped up, but can be used in conjunction with an epidural that can be topped up
Awareness and sensation	You are awake, but numb from the ribcage down, often including loss of feeling to legs
Set-up time	Can be set up in less than 10 minutes
Effect on the baby	Little effect on the baby
Implications for partner	Your partner or birth supporter can usually be present
Breastfeeding and skin contact	You can breastfeed and achieve 'skin-to-skin' contact immediately after the birth
Side-effects	Can lower blood pressure, make skin itchy, and cause nausea. Treatments are available to try to deal with all of these
Recovery	Can take 2–3 hours to completely wear off

Epidural	General anaesthetic
Anaesthetic given through a fine flexible tube into your spinal column	Anaesthetic given by cannula into your hand or arm. Gases given through a tube into your throat, once you are asleep
Can be topped up	Given continually until the operation is completed
You are awake, but numb from the ribcage down, often including loss of feeling to legs	You are asleep and unaware of any part of the operation
Can take half an hour or more to set up and take effect, but may be topped up in as little as 10 minutes, if already in place during labour	Can be achieved in less than 5 minutes and in a real emergency, can sometimes be the only option
Little effect on the baby	Can sometimes make the baby sleepy, floppy and occasionally have breathing problems
Your partner or birth supporter can usually be present	Your partner or birth supporter is not usually present
You can breastfeed and achieve 'skin-to-skin' contact immediately after the birth	Breastfeeding and contact with the baby are often delayed until you are fully awake
Can lower blood pressure, make skin itchy, and cause nausea. Treatments are available to try to deal with all of these	Can leave you with a congested chest and sore throat
Can take 6–8 hours to completely wear off	Can take several hours to be fully alert

If you would like more information about your anaesthetic choices, regardless as to whether a caesarean is booked, you can ask for an appointment with an anaesthetist.

Epidural

An epidural delivers anaesthetic fluid to your spinal column through a fine flexible tube called a catheter. The catheter will be taped to your back so that the epidural can be topped up as you need it.

An epidural can take at least half an hour to set up and take effect. If an epidural is already in place it can be topped up quickly for use during an emergency operation (sometimes in as little as 10 minutes).

You will be numb from the ribcage down, but you will be awake and aware of noises and sensation. Occasionally pain relief is incomplete. If this happens, you may be able to try a spinal anaesthetic so that you can still be awake. If regional anaesthesia fails to work sufficiently, you can be given a general anaesthetic.

General anaesthetic

A general anaesthetic (GA) sends your whole body to sleep so that you feel nothing. It can be used if regional anaesthesia does not give adequate pain relief. Some women find the prospect of being awake too daunting. If you feel strongly that you do not want a regional anaesthetic, you may request a general anaesthetic. Few consultants let a partner come into the operating theatre when a GA is used.

You may need a general anaesthetic if you have:

- severe back problems
- very low blood pressure
- bleeding
- a blood clotting disorder.

"The first thing I really wasn't expecting was how long the epidural took to set up. My husband thought they had forgotten him and had to ask a midwife to check if they had started without him. It would have been nice to know this, as we were already in a very stressful situation."

"I chose a general anaesthetic as I was concerned about being fully awake for the surgery. My husband remained with me through surgery and was able to tell me all the details and seemed to have thoroughly enjoyed the experience of being present."

General anaesthetic is given by cannula (a needle-like tube) into your hand or arm, and sends you to sleep in less than five minutes. You will be given oxygen and possibly more anaesthetic through a tube, which will be put into your throat once you are asleep. This is known as intubation.

If you use a name other than the name on your records, tell the staff before your operation so that afterwards they can wake you by the name you recognise.

Can I still make a birth plan?

It is helpful to think in advance and talk to your partner about what you might want to do if you have a caesarean. Then discuss your wishes with your obstetrician and midwife, and make a note of any agreements on a piece of paper headed 'birth preferences' or on your case notes. Make sure that both you and the hospital have a copy.

Although a caesarean section is a surgical operation, there are many choices and decisions you and your partner can make. Try to be fully involved in the decision to have a caesarean. Women who understand the need for their caesarean are less likely to feel depressed or upset afterwards than women who feel unsure and under pressure.

If you are not satisfied with the advice you have been given, you might want to find out more. You have a right to seek a second medical opinion. You may also change your consultant or hospital, even in late pregnancy.

When considering your preferences, there are a number of options to consider and arrangements you can make to make sure that the birth is a really special occasion for you and your partner.

You can find out more about caesarean birth and your options by:

● further reading

● internet research

● contacting the support organisations listed at the back of this booklet.

17

Ask your midwife or local antenatal teacher what the usual options and procedures are at your local hospitals. Hospital policies usually reflect the preferences of the lead obstetrician and can vary widely. Hospital trusts may also be worried about litigation and insurance issues. You can negotiate changes and you have a right to refuse interventions.

Options to consider

Anaesthetic: There are three types of anaesthetic (for more information, see *Can I choose my anaesthetic?* page 13). You should be offered an appointment with an anaesthetist to discuss your anaesthetic options.

Date and time: The NICE caesarean guideline recommends that planned caesareans are carried out after 39 weeks, because research shows that few babies born by caesarean after 39 weeks have breathing difficulties.[1]

Birth partners: Birth partners may usually be present if you are to be awake for the operation. If you have a general anaesthetic, it is unusual to have a partner with you, but in some hospitals partners may be allowed to stay and be first to hold the baby after he or she has been checked over.

If your partner is not allowed in, you may want to ask if it is possible for him or her to be nearby, possibly outside the theatre door. Your partner can then be told quickly when the baby is born and, if the baby is well, hold him/her soon afterwards.

Fathers who feel uncomfortable about being in theatre need not feel pressurised to attend. You may wish to ask someone else, such as a friend, relative or 'doula'. A doula is a paid, trained and experienced birth supporter (see page 78 for details).

Photographs: You may like to ask if it is possible for a member of staff or your birth supporter to take photographs of your baby at birth.

Mothers who have had a general anaesthetic have found a photograph of the baby being lifted out particularly precious. A small number of parents have been allowed to use video cameras.

Special care: If your baby needs to go to special care, you may like to consider whether you would prefer your partner to stay with you or to go with the baby.

If you have two people with you, you may want one to be with you and one with the baby. There may be a delay in admitting the baby's supporter to the special care unit while the baby is settled.

Multiple birth: if you are having more than one baby, you may want to ask to have your partner with you, plus one birth supporter for each of the babies.

Intensive Care Unit (ICU): If you go to intensive care because of pre-eclampsia or massive blood loss, then you may not be able to meet your baby for several hours or even days.

You may like to consider who you want to see your baby before you do. Some mothers have found it distressing that other members of their family were able to greet the new arrival before they were well enough to do so.

"I asked for my two birth partners to be present in theatre. At first, I was only allowed the father, but after some more discussion both were allowed in."

How can we make the birth special?

You may be surprised by the range of options available, even though a caesarean is surgery. Women who have had the chance before the birth to think about what is important to them have often found it helpful in making choices at the time.

Your options may include:

- a midwife to give a running commentary
- quiet in theatre, particularly at the moment of birth
- to have photographs taken
- to video the birth
- to watch the operation
- to use a mirror so that you can watch your baby being born
- to sit up a little, so you can see your baby being born
- for your baby to be delivered on to your chest
- to lift the baby out yourself
- for the lights to be dimmed at the moment of birth
- to be the first person to greet your baby
- to discover your baby's sex for yourself
- to have the baby resuscitation unit and weighing scales in sight
- to delay having your baby washed, bathed or dressed until you are back on the maternity ward and have fed him or her for the first time

"Caroline was using the video camera but inadvertently pressed the button back to standby mode at the wrong moment!"

- to have your baby with you in the recovery room so that you can start to breastfeed

- to be shown your placenta and have it explained to you by a midwife

- your partner, birth supporter or a known midwife to be the person to introduce your baby to you when you come round from a general anaesthetic.

In the operating theatre, there will be a screen, which prevents you from seeing what is happening. If you want to watch the operation, ask to have the screen lowered – or removed altogether – either for the whole operation or at the point of birth.

Health professionals may be wary of discussing caesarean preferences until they realise these are not medical requests, but environmental ones.

"Within minutes I was laid down, fully numb from the waist down, hooked up to all the machines and our music CD was playing in the background. The consultant asked if we would like to have the screen high or low and said that she would be starting very soon. We had the screen low so my husband could peer over and see what was happening."

"Just before Catherine was about to be delivered the consultant asked if we would like the screen lowered completely. I was then able to raise my head up and see her lifted out of me and lowered onto my chest. I cuddled her and wondered at how much vernix she was covered in and thought how amazing she was."

About the operation

What will happen before my caesarean?

If your caesarean is planned, you will be asked to go into hospital early on the day of the operation or the night before. You will be asked not to eat or drink after a certain time so that your stomach is empty at the time of the operation.

If it is expected that your baby may need to go into the special care baby unit (SCBU), you can usually visit the unit before the birth. There may be a leaflet or video about the unit. Many women find it comforting to know where their babies are if they are not able to visit them immediately after the birth.

You will usually be given a time for your operation but it may be delayed by emergency cases or lack of postnatal beds. A delay can be difficult to cope with, especially if it happens more than once.

Women express many different emotions about the waiting time leading up to the operation. These include worry, excitement, boredom and fear.

It may be helpful to plan how you and your birth partner will spend the time. Other parents have passed this time by:

- using relaxation or massage techniques
- reassuring their baby with words or positive thoughts
- listening to music

"We arrived early at the hospital – a very understanding nurse admitted me and prepared me for theatre. She had taken the time to read my notes and arranged for me to be the first of the three electives that morning so I wouldn't have to wait any longer than necessary. It was much appreciated. But other emergencies meant theatre was busy and I didn't make the nervous walk to theatre until 2.30pm."

- reading newspapers, magazines or books

- playing cards or board games.

You will be asked to sign a consent form. Without this legal document, surgery can be considered assault. Before you sign the form, you should have an opportunity to talk to your doctor to make sure you understand what will be happening to you and your baby – the reasons why, and any possible complications.

For safety, you will be asked to take off:

- jewellery (your wedding ring may be taped over)

- glasses or contact lenses (but keep your glasses handy as you will normally be able to use them to see your baby during the operation)

- hair clips

- make-up and nail polish (so that the anaesthetist can monitor your colouring)

- removable brace or false teeth.

You will change into a hospital gown, which is open at the back. You may be wheeled to theatre on a trolley, with a blanket over you for warmth and modesty; or you may walk into theatre and get on to the operating table.

Your birth partner will have to wear theatre clothes, and possibly theatre footwear and a mask. You may not recognise them at first!

You may be given an antacid. This is a medicine given by mouth to neutralise stomach acid and so reduce the risk in the unlikely event of vomiting under general anaesthetic.

"I felt and saw our second son being born. Who says it's not as good as the 'real thing'? It's wonderful. Don't knock it if you haven't tried it."

"He looked great in two-inches-above-the-ankle length white trousers, a blue top to fit a 36" female, a blue cloth tied over his head and a dust mask round his nose and mouth.
I hope the photo the anaesthetist took comes out."

"Although my glasses were removed, I did get them back once my baby was born so I was able to see her properly."

A sample of your blood is taken to check for anaemia and sometimes to check for your blood group. In rare cases of heavy bleeding or severe anaemia you may need a blood transfusion.

The area where the scar will be, usually across the top of the pubic hair, may be shaved. The skin is swabbed with antiseptic, which may be bright orange.

You will need a catheter (a thin plastic tube) inserted into your bladder to keep it empty. Some women do not feel the catheter at all, while others find it painful when it is being put in. If you are having spinal or epidural anaesthetic, the catheter can usually be inserted after the anaesthetic starts to work.

The midwife may fit you with some white stockings or pneumatic boots that feel tight and warm. They are to help avoid DVT (deep vein thrombosis) or blood clots. You will usually be asked to keep these on until you are out of bed again. Sometimes heparin injections are used instead of stockings. Heparin is a drug used to thin the blood and prevent clots from forming.

The operating table is tilted or wedged to the left. This relieves the pressure of the uterus on the vena cava, the major blood vessel taking blood back to the heart, and helps to prevent a fall in blood pressure.

An intravenous (IV) drip feeds fluid into a vein, usually on the back of your hand or arm. This can be used to maintain blood pressure, and helps if you need drugs during the operation.

A blood pressure cuff on your arm may be operated automatically and tightened from time to time.

"I was not prepared for all the monitoring equipment – oxygen mask, catheter, blood pressure monitor. I felt like a very large, immobile alien."

"Although I was very scared during the operation, we had the radio on and the staff did their best to relax me, and I'm sure I would have been scared with a normal delivery. At least with a caesarean I knew it would be over in a relatively short amount of time, and that I wouldn't be exhausted before I had the baby, even though I certainly was afterwards!"

Electrodes attached to your chest monitor your heart rate and you may have a finger pulse monitor. This is a bit like a thimble and is painless.

A sticky plastic plate is attached to your leg. This is part of the equipment that the surgeon uses to seal the blood vessels.

You may be given oxygen through a mask – this can help the baby if fetal distress is suspected.

Who will be there?

You may be surprised how crowded the operating theatre or labour room is during a caesarean section. There could be as many as 16 unknown people in cases of multiple birth or if the baby is believed to be at risk. There are unlikely to be fewer than six staff.

For the mother, there may be:

- a midwife

- the consultant obstetrician or registrar who operates

- surgeon's assistant

- an anaesthetist

- the scrub nurse

- an anaesthetic nurse or operating department assistant (ODA)

- a theatre/running nurse

- an interpreter, if the woman is deaf or her first language isn't English.

For the baby, there may be:

- a midwife

"I found the number of people in theatre very frightening. I didn't know who half of them were or why they were there. I wish I had had the courage to ask them all to either leave or to be silent so that I could greet my baby the way I had planned."

"We got into the theatre and there were people everywhere! It was scary as I had had the romantic notion that it was going to be like my first birth – me, my husband and two midwives! I know with twins there has to be extra staff but 22! I freaked and had a general. If I had been warned about how many people would be in theatre and that they do indeed all have a role to do, I would have been braver."

- a paediatrician. If the caesarean is elective, and there is no concern about the baby's well being, a paediatrician may not be present
- If the baby is believed to be at risk, there will also be a paediatric resuscitation team, with an incubator.

Medical students or student midwives may be observing. You should be asked if you mind students being present. You are entitled to ask that students are not present.

Will I feel the operation?

The effectiveness of regional anaesthetic varies, and will be tested, often with a cold liquid, ice or a pinprick to ensure women feel no pain during the operation. Some mothers experience a sensation that they liken to having a pencil drawn across the abdomen. Feelings of tugging and pulling when the baby is born are very common.

If you are asleep under a general anaesthetic, you will not be aware that the operation is taking place. However, the anaesthetic is light, and very occasionally women report a vague awareness.

In extremely rare cases, women have felt pain under general anaesthetic, but have been unable to communicate this to the anaesthetist. Precautions are now taken to avoid this.

How long does it take?

For a first caesarean, it can take as little as five to ten minutes until the baby is born, although the whole operation can take up to an hour or more. If it is a second or subsequent caesarean it can take longer due to the presence of scar tissue from previous operations.

"I started to feel a rummaging and yanking in my tummy. It felt as though someone had opened a door at a jumble sale and a free-for-all was going on."

"Once surgery was under way, I had no idea at all how much pulling and tugging you could still feel, although totally painless, it was an extremely odd situation to be in and I was unprepared for that."

26

What happens during a caesarean?

It is usual for a screen to be placed over the mother's chest, which prevents her from seeing the operation, although some parents have asked for this to be lowered at the moment of birth.

There is a large light above the operating table, in which some women have seen an unclear mirror image of the operation. For some this is quite disconcerting, while others find it reassuring.

The obstetrician cuts through the various layers of tissue, pulls the abdominal muscles aside, and gently moves the bladder away from the wall of the uterus. Then an incision is made in the uterus through which the baby is born (see *Where will I have a scar?* page 44).

Different surgeons will use different surgical techniques, and these may vary depending on individual circumstances. A wound drain may be inserted if necessary.

Occasionally women who have used epidural or spinal anaesthesia have reported retching or being sick during the operation. You can be given drugs or acupressure to prevent or treat this.

Some women have been asked to help push their babies out by contracting their muscles. If you put your hand on your chest, you may be able to feel your baby move down. The surgeon doing the operation will probably lift the baby out, sometimes using forceps. At one hospital mothers have been allowed to lift out their baby themselves.

Breech babies are delivered bottom first, and, if you are having twins, the lower twin (twin 1) is born first.

"About 10 minutes into the operation, all the staff there who were not immediately busy, also stood almost to attention with rapt expressions of awe on their faces. They were all looking towards my stomach and I realised that something momentous was happening, I had no idea that the birth would be so soon after arriving in the theatre. I have never forgotten the look of reverence on their faces at the moment of the birth; that team must have done loads of similar operations yet they all seemed as proud and delighted as though it was their own baby."

Your new baby

What happens to my baby?

Usually the newborn baby is handed to a midwife or a paediatrician to be examined, but some babies are placed on their mother's chest. You may ask to be the first to discover the sex of your baby. All babies have their condition assessed at one and five minutes after birth. This is recorded as an Apgar score. A normal baby in good condition will have an Apgar score between 7 and 10. The maximum score at each assessment is 10.

The baby is rated from 0–2 on each of five items:

- heart rate
- breathing
- muscle tone
- reflexes
- colour.

If all is well, you or your partner should be able to hold your baby while you are stitched. You should also all be able to be together afterwards in the recovery room.

All newborn babies are weighed and washed, although this need not be done immediately. You may enjoy watching your baby being bathed, reading the weight for yourself, and taking photographs later, when you are back on the ward.

If you have a general anaesthetic, it is usually possible for your birth partner to hold the baby, and to introduce him or her to you when you wake up.

Women who labour before a caesarean may feel that the labour was pointless, and that they put their baby at risk. However, evidence shows that contractions are important as they prepare the baby's lungs for breathing.[14]

Babies whose mothers have not been through labour before their caesarean are more likely to have respiratory distress at birth and later respiratory problems than babies whose mothers laboured before their caesarean. If your baby is in difficulties before the caesarean section, you will be given oxygen through a mask before the birth. Some babies will need help to start or maintain breathing.

Parents and midwives have noted that some babies seem shocked or angry at the speed of their birth, others are calm.

Some caesarean babies are noted for their 'perfect-looking' round heads that have not been moulded by passage through the birth canal.

Some babies may be bruised or have marks due to their position in the uterus or experiences during birth and occasionally babies can be cut by the surgeon's scalpel.

Can I have 'skin-to-skin' contact with my baby?

In many units 'skin-to-skin' contact is encouraged soon after your baby is born. You hold your baby, who is wearing nothing, or only a nappy, against your body. Your baby can get to know you using all his or her senses. This is comforting and can help get breastfeeding off to a good start. It can be a lovely way to welcome your new baby however you decide to feed.

"I was surprised how bloody he was and he came out screaming in anger at being disturbed from his nice cosy warm sleep! He looked at us all in such disgust. I was amazed at how his colour changed as well. I was expecting the bluey, purple colour, but didn't realise how quickly a baby 'pinks up'."

"I am amazed how within 40 minutes of such intense feelings of fear, and major surgery, I was laying in recovery with my perfect little baby girl, breastfeeding her. Listening to her make little noises and feeling her on the outside of my body rather than within. It's a truly remarkable experience."

'Skin-to-skin' can also prevent babies from becoming chilled and is a good way of warming a cold baby. Theatre gowns can often make this difficult. If your baby needs special care, 'skin-to-skin' contact or kangaroo care may still be possible.

If you would like 'skin-to-skin' contact with your baby, discuss it with your midwife so that preparations can be made. Some fathers also enjoy 'skin-to-skin' contact with their babies.

Will my baby need special care?

Some babies, especially those born prematurely, need to go to a special care baby unit (SCBU) after they are born. They may need help with breathing or feeding, and their condition in the early days may need to be monitored regularly.

If your baby needs special care, it can be invaluable to have a second supporter so that both mother and baby can benefit from close emotional support, and the mother can be told in detail about the baby's early hours and progress.

If your hospital does not provide the level of care your baby needs, he or she may need to be transferred by ambulance to a more specialist neonatal intensive care unit (NICU). If it is known in advance that your baby may need intensive care you may be transferred to a more specialist unit before your baby's birth. This may also happen if the SCBU in your hospital is full or does not have sufficient staff. Sometimes babies have to be taken a long distance to the nearest available cot with suitable care facilities.

"It all happened so suddenly. What had seemed to be a normal progressing labour became an emergency...and our lives were changed forever."

SCBU: Special care baby unit

NICU: Neonatal intensive care unit

Kangaroo care: Keeping your baby inside your clothes (skin-to-skin) can have positive effects for special care babies.

Managed clinical networks are being introduced to try to ensure that parents and doctors can know in advance which specialist unit babies would be referred to if additional care was needed.

It may not be possible for your partner or supporter to be present while your baby is admitted to the unit. There may not be enough space, or there may be urgent procedures to carry out. For example, the staff may be concerned that insertion of drips may be distressing. Visitors should be welcome once the baby is stable.

Depending on space, and the local health and safety policy, it may not be possible for the father to travel in an ambulance with the baby. If he is to go with his baby, he may need someone else to drive him, rather than drive himself at such a stressful time.

If there is more than one baby, each baby's needs will be assessed individually. This can occasionally mean that the babies are cared for in different units.

Mothers often have to stay at the hospital where they had the baby for several days. Parents face the agonising decision: does the partner stay with the mother or go with the baby?

Can I breastfeed my baby?

A caesarean should not alter a mother's choice of the way she feeds her baby. A caesarean should not normally affect a woman's ability to produce milk. However, you may find it more difficult to sit or lie comfortably and you may need to experiment with positions to avoid pressure or strain on the wound.

Breastmilk is the ideal food for your baby. It contains everything your baby needs to eat and drink for the first six months, and helps protect your baby from infections and other illness.

"I was given a general anaesthetic and my baby was delivered 10 minutes later with an Apgar of 4 rising to 7 at five minutes. He was transferred to the neonatal unit at the district hospital about seven miles away before I'd come round from the anaesthetic."

"I remained in hospital for nearly two weeks; I would have been discharged after five days if my baby had not been in the neonatal unit and I had not lived so far away."

"The midwife in recovery helped my baby to attach to my breast. It helped to take away some of the emotional pain of the operation."

Many women lose confidence in their mothering abilities after a caesarean or other assisted birth, and support for simple day-to-day tasks may be in short supply. Do ask for help when you need it.

Women who have had a caesarean may be especially determined to make breastfeeding work. Some mothers find it useful to talk through their feelings with a trained breastfeeding counsellor.

A few mothers have managed to breastfeed in the operating theatre, but it is more usual for the first feed to take place in the recovery room or on the postnatal ward.

If you, or your baby, are not well, the first breastfeed may be delayed for many hours. If this happens, your baby may not be as eager to feed as would be expected in the first hour or so after birth. 'Skin-to-skin' contact, cuddles, and plenty of patience are the best remedy.

If you want to breastfeed your baby, tell your carers. Formula milk is rarely necessary for breastfed babies and can undermine successful breastfeeding.

If you think you might want to breastfeed, remember that it is easier to change from breastfeeding to bottle feeding with formula than to change the other way around.

If you give your baby formula milk, you will make less breastmilk. If your baby needs more milk, try feeding more often (rather than giving formula milk).

At first, you will produce colostrum, which is small in quantity but full of valuable antibodies that will protect your baby from infection. Colostrum provides all the nutrition your baby needs for the first few days.

The time taken for the milk to change from colostrum varies from mother to mother. Although some caesarean mothers report that their milk is slow to come in, women who have had vaginal births also report this.

You and your baby are learning a new skill when starting to breastfeed, and recovery from a caesarean means that you have additional difficulties to overcome.

Some women find the wound a problem when they are trying to get comfortable to feed and the baby may be capable of a well-directed kick! The caesarean may mean that you are unable to sit as you normally would. Many women experience backache.

At first, it may be most comfortable to lie down to feed. You will need someone to bring your baby to you. In this position, your baby lies beside you, so that you can rest, or even sleep, while you feed. If you are sitting, it helps to support yourself with pillows or cushions, particularly if you are still on a drip. It can also help to use a pillow to support your baby.

Many women find they get a better latch if they position their baby first and pack in cushions to support the baby, rather than trying to balance the baby on a cushion.

Holding your baby 'chest to chest' will help to get a good breastfeeding position while avoiding pressure on the wound. You may need to experiment with positions and find what is comfortable for you and avoids putting pressure on the wound. When you sit in a chair or on the side of a bed, if your feet do not easily reach the floor, you may find it helpful to use a footrest – a box or a pile of large books will do.

"I felt I had missed out on a normal birth, and wanted to breastfeed to prove that my body could get something right."

"Being laid flat on my back, I could just see the top of his head as he was feeding. It was just the most wonderful thing I had ever seen. He knew just what to do and latched on straight away."

"The staff were really great at helping me get comfortable in readiness to feed Matthew."

Sometimes painkillers can mask the pain of sore nipples. If you notice your nipples look sore, even though they do not feel it, talk to your midwife or breastfeeding counsellor. This problem is often due to poor positioning or thrush (a fungal infection).

What drugs affect breastfeeding?

Most drugs taken for pain relief are compatible with breastfeeding. If you have any worries about drugs affecting your baby, talk to your midwife, breastfeeding counsellor or paediatrician.

Some drugs given for maternal conditions such as pre-eclampsia, blood clotting or thyroid disorders may be incompatible with breastfeeding. There may be alternatives, so discuss this with your carers or a breastfeeding counsellor.

If you will be taking such a medication for only a short time, you may want to express your milk and discard it. This may help you keep up your milk supply until it is safe to establish breastfeeding. Your baby may be able to be given donated breastmilk from a milk bank, if there is one operating locally.

My baby is in special care. Can I breastfeed?

If your baby has to go to SCBU or NICU you should still be able to give him or her breastmilk. Your colostrum will be of special value to your special care baby, as it will protect the lining of the intestine and give immunity from many infections, including some which can be life threatening.

If you cannot feed your baby directly, or if he or she is not being given milk at first, someone should show you how to hand express your milk. You can use this as the only method of expressing or to start the milk flowing before you use a breast pump. Colostrum is thick and produced in small quantities. When using a pump, it sticks to the insides of tubes and beakers. Hand expressing may be particularly useful in collecting this valuable milk.

At first, your baby may be given breastmilk through a tube. Later, your baby can be fed expressed breastmilk from a small cup, spoon or syringe. If you use a bottle too early, it can confuse a young baby, which may make it difficult for him or her to learn to breastfeed.

If your baby cannot have your milk to begin with, you can freeze the expressed milk for future use. Regular expressing, including at night, to mimic a baby's feeding pattern, will help to maintain your milk supply for your baby. Short, frequent sessions of expressing are better than long sessions less often.

Although the large electric pumps are most efficient at expressing milk, you can get hand, battery and smaller electric pumps that are more portable. There is further information in the NCT leaflet *Breastfeeding: how to express and store your milk* (details on page 75).

Can I choose to bottle feed my baby?

A caesarean should not alter a mother's choice of the way she feeds her baby and some mothers prefer to bottle feed.

If you are planning to bottle feed, you may want to discuss who is going to give the first feed, and when and where this will be done.

Information on all aspects of bottle feeding is available from midwives and health visitors. You may

"I did use a breast pump, it was good for reassuring the doctors that he had had a good fluid intake. I found it a bit mechanical, but had no problems providing the gold top."

You can find out more about breastfeeding and feeding your baby expressed milk in the NCT leaflets *Breastfeeding – a good start* and *Breastfeeding – how to express and store your milk*, details on page 75.

35

also like to contact other mothers who have bottle fed after a caesarean. See page 75 to find your nearest NCT branch.

If you begin by breastfeeding, but decide later on that you would prefer to switch to bottle feeding, you can find help and support from breastfeeding organisations (see pages 75-79) or from your midwife or health visitor.

Early recovery

What happens to me after my baby is born?

After your baby is born, your placenta is removed through the caesarean incision. You will be given an injection of syntometrine or syntocinon (see right) via a drip. Occasionally, women using regional anaesthesia have reported discomfort during this stage.

The 'closing up' stage usually takes longer than the previous stages. There are two main sets of stitches. The incision in the uterus is repaired with soluble stitches usually using a double layer technique, although some surgeons now use a single layer closure (see *Will I have stitches?* on page 43).

The second set of stitches closes the skin of the abdomen (see *What will my scar be like?* on page 45).

Where will I go after theatre?

After the operation, you will probably be taken to the post-operative recovery room, or a labour ward room, so your condition can be monitored before you are transferred to the postnatal ward. You can usually have your birth partner(s) with you at this time.

When you first come round after a general anaesthetic, a nurse or midwife should reassure you that all is well and explain where you are. You may feel detached and drowsy, and drift in and out of sleep. It can be dreamlike, and your memory of this time may be hazy.

Syntocinon and syntometrine are drugs that:

- help the uterus to contract
- close the blood vessels which supplied the placenta
- reduce the risk of postpartum haemorrhage (excessive loss of blood – more than 500ml – from the uterus after the baby is born)

Often mothers meet their baby as they come round from the anaesthetic. Some appreciate the birth partner – rather than someone they do not know – introducing the baby. Many women say that photographs have helped to reinforce their memory of their first meeting.

If all is well, you will then be taken to the postnatal ward. Depending on availability, and the needs of other mothers, you may be offered a single room. If you have a preference, it is worth discussing this with the midwives. Sometimes you may be able to pay for a separate amenity room.

You may appreciate privacy and quiet, or you may prefer the company of other mothers on the main ward, and the more frequent interaction with staff. It may be helpful to talk to other mothers who have had a caesarean.

Whatever type of room you are in, you should have a call bell that you can reach easily and without discomfort. Caesarean mothers need more help – don't feel guilty about using your call bell as often as you need.

In rare cases, such as severe pre-eclampsia, it is possible you may come round on the intensive care ward. A nurse will probably wake you by calling your name and telling you where you are. Depending on your condition, you may be wired up to equipment and could have drips in both arms.

Your first meeting with your baby may be delayed but if your baby is well, he or she should be brought to you. Many mothers find this separation very difficult to deal with, and the sadness may remain with them long after the event.

"I came round about 20 minutes later, back in my room, and I couldn't stop crying and saying 'I'm sorry'. Benjamin was handed to me fully clothed, which was something I had wanted to avoid, as I had really wanted to see my baby as a newborn – with no clothes, straight from my tummy. I was depressed for a long time and for the first six months of his life I really felt he could have belonged to anybody."

Photographs and regular reports from staff and family can help keep you in touch with your baby and some hospitals have a video link to SCBU.

Will I be in pain afterwards?

Although a caesarean is often seen as a 'pain free' form of birth, it is major surgery, so you will be offered treatment for post-surgical pain.

If you have had a regional anaesthetic it will provide pain relief for some time after the operation. A spinal can take 2–3 hours to wear off while an epidural will often last longer – it could take 6–8 hours for the effects to wear off completely.

On waking up from a general anaesthetic you should already have been given pain relief, although occasionally women have reported pain on waking.

There are many post-caesarean pain relief options so you may want to find out what is available at your hospital. You may also want to ask how and when pain medication is normally given.

Some of the options include:

- epidural – sometimes drugs for pain relief in the immediate post-surgical recovery period may be given through the epidural before it is removed

- intravenous (IV) drip – drugs can be given using the intravenous drip you had for the caesarean itself

- patient-controlled anaesthetic (PCA) – this can be attached to the IV by the anaesthetist before you leave theatre. You control the amount of drug yourself by pressing a button

"The length of time for final twinges of pain to disappear and for tenderness at the scar to go surprised me, about nine months for the first and up to a year for the second caesarean."

"When I arrived on the ward, I was offered a self-administered morphine drip which was hooked up to my IV. The morphine drip was excellent because I was in control of how much drug I was putting into my system. It allowed me to press a button whenever I felt I needed to 'top up' my pain relief. The morphine was effective enough even though I kept the dosage low (as I wanted to breastfeed and I was a little worried about passing on the morphine to my newborn)."

- injections – may be given to take over when the spinal/epidural wears off

- suppositories (inserted into your rectum) – can be inserted in theatre or given postnatally on the ward

- oral (by mouth) – tablets, capsules, liquid

- TENS (transcutaneous nerve stimulation) machine – does not use drugs. It gives tiny electrical pulses to the skin around the wound.

A variety of drugs may be used. Some of the more common include:

- opiates such as morphine, diamorphine (heroin), codeine, pethidine, meptazinol (Meptid)

- non-steroidal anti-inflammatory drugs such as ibuprofen or diclofenac (eg Voltarol)

- non-opioid drugs such as paracetamol

- combinations such as paracetamol with codeine, ibuprofen, or diclophenac.

The type of pain relief you will be offered may depend on the circumstances of your caesarean, your general health, the amount and type of drugs you have already been given, and what is usual at the hospital. Most drugs used for pain relief following caesarean are compatible with breastfeeding.

Some drugs take effect quickly but provide pain relief for a short period, while others take longer to start giving relief but are effective for many hours.

Dosages and length of time of adequate pain relief will vary according to your weight, your individual response to the drug given, and the amount of pain you are in.

Side effects are common, particularly with opioid drugs. They may include constipation, nausea, vomiting, drowsiness and disorientation. If you are concerned about your reactions, discuss them with the midwives and doctors caring for you.

Postnatal wards are often busy and sometimes short staffed so if you are in pain – do speak up. Most women find it is better to take painkillers regularly to keep on top of the pain and many have found it helpful to be aware of when their next medication is due. It may also take time for staff to organise this.

If you try to be 'brave', you may end up in more pain, be less mobile, and so less able to look after your baby. If your pain builds up, it may be more difficult to achieve an adequate level of pain relief and you may need a larger dose of the drug.

Pain relief may mean you do not notice developing aches and pains, such as backache and sore nipples. Extra care needs to be taken with posture, especially when sitting or moving. The same applies when positioning the baby at the breast, if you are breastfeeding.

Many women progress quite quickly to taking paracetamol only. If you feel the pain relief is not strong enough, or not given often enough, discuss this with the midwives caring for you.

If you have any concerns, or want information on which drugs are used, you can ask for a consultation to discuss your options with a midwife, doctor or anaesthetist. You can do this either before or after your caesarean.

If you have learned relaxation skills or other self-help methods for coping with pain in preparation for the birth, you may find them useful now. They can be

"I had received a really good pre-op chat from the anaesthetist who had told me to 'keep on top of the pain' by taking pain relief pre-emptively for the first week. He said that if you think 'I am brave, I can take a bit of pain', you will suffer unnecessarily. There is medical evidence to suggest that once you have let your pain come through, it is then harder to overcome it again with painkillers. I actually agreed with him 100%."

especially useful when you have any medical procedures done (for example having stitches or drains removed) or when you stand up or move.

When might it hurt most?

Although the pain is usually kept under control by medication, there are situations when it can be particularly noticeable. Changing positions in bed, getting in and out of bed and moving around can hurt at first.

You may find it hurts most when you laugh or cough. It often helps to hold a pillow over your wound to support it. Do not suppress the need to cough, particularly after a general anaesthetic, as it is important to keep your lungs clear.

Some women find they need to pass wind frequently after a caesarean. Post-operative wind may also cause discomfort and pain in the abdomen and elsewhere in the body – even in the shoulders. Some women find peppermint helps.

You may also experience pain or discomfort in the perineal area (see *Will I bleed afterwards?* opposite) as a result of procedures such as vaginal examinations, fetal blood sampling or a failed forceps delivery. A few women also have perineal stitches.

Some women find they are left with bruising or soreness where the drip was inserted.

An obstetric physiotherapist may visit you to suggest exercises and show you how to move more easily. This information may be provided on printed sheets or in a leaflet.

"I had no hesitation in asking for pain relief from the hospital staff as it became due, even if they had not offered it yet (after all, they get busy and cannot monitor exactly how long since your last dose!)"

"I found it really hard as it really hurt when I laughed, so I had to tell my husband to stop trying to cheer me up!"

"The worst thing about the whole experience was the wind. It caused me more pain than the section ever did."

Will I bleed afterwards?

Some caesarean mothers are surprised that they bleed, but in this respect they are no different from women who have given birth vaginally. Lochia is a natural discharge of blood that helps to clear the uterus. At first it is deep red and rather like a heavy period. It gradually becomes paler. Some women discharge clots of blood with the lochia. Small clots are normal. If you are worried, discuss this with your midwife.

Will I have stitches?

In the case of the usual bikini line cut you will have a skin wound about 15–22cms (6–9ins) long, generally on a horizontal line in your upper pubic hair, covered by a dressing.

The wound is commonly closed by a running stitch with a bead at each end, although other methods include staples or clips. Sometimes dissolving stitches are used which will not require removal. Some women have reported allergic reactions to the metal in the clips or staples.

The internal tissue will be stitched with dissolving stitches, which you may notice discharged with the lochia (see above).

Occasionally you may also have a tube or 'drain' from the abdomen to drain off excess fluid from the wound. The fluid may be a thick, dark, bloody colour.

After washing your wound, pat it dry with a clean towel or paper towel. Using a hair dryer is not recommended.

Some women find complementary therapies helpful with healing.

"Having had metal clips the first time, which had taken ages to remove, the running stitch with beads was quite a relief."

"I was surprised when the running stitch was taken out as I hardly felt it – a friend had warned me it really hurt."

"I remember being quite shocked at the sight of metal clips staring up at me. I'd sort of expected just stitches."

A midwife will usually remove your stitches or clips around five days after the caesarean, depending on your consultant's preference. You may be able to negotiate the timing.

Some women find the removal of stitches only slightly uncomfortable, while others feel pain. You can ask for painkillers, and relaxation techniques can be extremely helpful.

You can ask to look at or keep beads, thread, clips or staples.

Where will I have a scar?

Inside, on the uterus

The most common uterine incision used today is the lower segment caesarean section (LSCS), which is horizontal.

LSCS is preferred because it heals more quickly and gives a stronger scar. This incision rarely causes problems for future pregnancies.

Vertical uterine incisions include:

- lower midline vertical: a vertical cut in the uterus, sometimes used for delivering premature babies, when the lower segment of the uterus may not be sufficiently developed
- inverted T or J incisions – the names describe the shape
- classical – the original large vertical caesarean incision type which is now rarely used.

Outside, on the skin

Occasionally the type of incision you have outside on your skin will be different from the one on your

"The scar area remained sensitive for about 4–6 weeks, but was not so painful that I had to take anything for it after the first 10 days. Now, a year later, I still have the occasional twinge on the right side of my scar, but nothing major."

"Four months after my caesarean I still have numbness and pain in the scar area. I'm going back to my GP about that."

uterus. Nowadays, the skin cut is usually a horizontal one, just below the pubic hairline, often called a bikini cut.

If a scar from a previous caesarean has not healed neatly, the surgeon can often tidy this up at the time of a subsequent caesarean.

What will my scar be like?

Until you get home, you may not have a chance to have a good look at your scar. Some women find themselves putting this off. A woman's body image may be very different after having a baby, particularly if she has a caesarean scar.

You may be anxious about the first time that your partner sees your scar, and he may be worried about it too. Most women find it helpful to discuss their feelings fully with their partner sooner rather than later.

The appearance of the scar can vary a great deal from woman to woman. To begin with, it is likely that it will look quite red, but this will fade over time, to something nearer your skin colour, that may be barely noticeable.

To see for yourself a range of scars, the website www.caesarean.org.uk has a collection of pictures that women, worldwide, have kindly agreed to share.

Scars may be smooth or lumpy, even or lopsided, straight or curved. Most are completely covered by the pubic hair.

Occasionally, a keloid scar may form as part of the scar tissue. This is a growth of fibrous tissue in a scar and is particularly common among black women.

"I hadn't realised how itchy my scar would be for months afterwards, and occasionally it does still get itchy."

"Although there seemed to be a lot of blood under the bandages of the wound, when it was cleaned up, the scar healed really well. I took arnica tablets which I'm convinced helped the healing process."

Keloid scars have been described as feeling lumpy and hard to the touch, like a hard ridge or bone. They can be tender, but are not always.

A common complaint among caesarean mothers is the way their tummies overhang their scars, although some women do retain a flat tummy. There seems to be little that women can do about this.

Many women find their scar sensitive, itchy or generally uncomfortable. Your pubic hair will start to re-grow after having been shaved for the operation, and the stubble can be very itchy. Numb patches on the scar and elsewhere are also common. There is usually improvement in the first few months but for some women these remain indefinitely.

Adhesions may also form. They are a normal response to surgery in which scar tissue forms that may cause abdominal organs or layers of tissue, which normally move freely, to bind together. These can occasionally cause discomfort and some women have reported feeling adhesions stretch or snap during subsequent pregnancies.

If you are unhappy or worried about the look or feel of your scar, you may want to consult your family doctor or your obstetrician. In severe cases, further surgery may be recommended.

Is there a risk of infection?

It is widely accepted that having a caesarean section greatly increases the risk of postnatal infection. Types of infection include: infections of the wound, urinary tract or bladder and uterine infections. Usually these are treatable with antibiotics although there are growing concerns about bacteria that are resistant

"I stopped using the public changing area of the swimming baths, and I wouldn't let my husband touch me near the scar. It certainly did not help my self image."

"For a long time, I had very little sensation on my tummy, but that seems to have largely returned (although not quite). Since my tummy always used to be a very sensitive zone, I wasn't best pleased that it had become so insensitive, and I have to say it's not quite the same as it used to be, alas."

to antibiotics, e.g. MRSA (methicillin-resistant *Staphylococcus aureus*).

Research has shown that antibiotics significantly reduce the incidence of wound infections.[17] These are usually given in a single dose by injection in theatre. If you suspect you may have problems with antibiotics, you may want to discuss this before the operation.

If you have any worries about your scar, particularly if it is inflamed or sore, mention this to your midwife or doctor straight away. If you have any other concerns or discomforts, it is as well to bring them to the attention of your midwife or doctor, so prompt treatment can be given if necessary.

In hospital, showering may be preferable to bathing. Normal hygiene at home will be adequate. Take extra care to avoid bringing the scar into contact with germs from other people's baths or towels.

Who should I ask about my operation?

If you have any questions about your operation, the labour you may have had beforehand, or your recovery, you should be able to go through your notes with one of the midwives. It may also be possible to talk with the midwife who cared for you.

Your obstetrician, or a registrar who will visit the ward, should also be able to give information about the operation and why it was necessary.

If you feel it would be useful, you can ask to see the person who did the caesarean section.

Some hospitals have printed information and we also list helpful organisations on page 75-79.

"I needed ongoing treatment for my infection. I remember travelling home from one of our trips to hospital, cradling Joe, blood and pus seeping onto my dress, thinking over and over, "I can't believe all this is happening to me."

Your hospital stay

How long will I be in hospital?

The length of your hospital stay will depend on hospital policy and your personal circumstances and preferences. It is usual to stay between 3–5 days. This is something to discuss with your carers.

You may want your visitors to come at different times during your stay, rather than all at once. Some women ask their partner or the midwives to explain that they do not yet feel up to being sociable, but would welcome a visit later.

Visits by the baby's older brothers or sisters may be a challenge, both emotionally and physically. Toddlers may not understand that you have just had an operation and they mustn't jump on your tummy.

You may like to think about how to protect your scar so you can cuddle your other children. For example, you could sit in a chair or cover the wound with a pillow. You may all feel sad when they have to go home and leave you in hospital.

What do I need in hospital?

To pack

Maternity sanitary pads: You need these to absorb the lochia (the vaginal bleeding that follows all births, see *Will I bleed afterwards?* on page 43).

Knickers: Caesarean mothers usually prefer high-waisted knickers that reach over the top of the scar, as bikini briefs can be very uncomfortable. It is best to avoid knickers made of nylon or lacy fabric as they can catch on or irritate stitches, scabs and pubic hair as it re-grows.

"With my third caesarean I felt confident to return home to my family the following day."

"The five days I spent in hospital were fine – but it was lovely to be home again."

"On the Friday (two days after the operation) I was allowed to go home, since I was obviously doing well, was not in pain and basically just wanted to get home with my partner and baby to start enjoying our parenthood."

48

Nightie: A short-sleeved nightie may be easier when coping with a drip and a warm hospital ward. Some silky materials make sitting more difficult as they tend to slip against pillows and bedclothes.

Slippers: Bending down may be awkward at first, so you may find slip-on slippers or bare feet easiest.

Drinking bottle or cup: Some women have found a bottle or cup with a lid useful until mobility improves and sitting upright is easier.

Mobility aids: If you use one, take in your own mobility aid, for example wheelchair, frame or crutches. It may be useful to check in advance that your needs will be met by the rooms and facilities on the postnatal ward.

NCT Sales (see page 75) are a good source of nighties and comfortable stretch knickers that dry easily and allow good air circulation to your healing wound.

To ask for

Stool or step: Getting in and out of bed can be a challenge. Most caesarean mothers are given height-adjustable beds. A small footstool can be very useful if you are in a non-adjustable bed.

Cots: You could also ask for an adjustable crib or clip-on cot. These are now available in many maternity units for use by disabled women and those having caesareans. They can make it easier for mothers to care for their babies, giving a greater degree of independence.

Pillows: Most hospitals will supply extra pillows, but you may have to ask, or you could bring in your own. You will find these help keep you comfortable and provide necessary support when you are feeding your baby.

"One of the best things I had were some really big pants ... ones that your Nan would be proud of. These were good because they came up and over the scar and didn't rub."

"None of the equipment was well designed for someone who had had major abdominal surgery. The beds were too high; there was only one adjustable height bed on the ward. There weren't even many stools. The light switches and call bell were out of reach. I had to lever myself painfully up inch by inch to reach them – getting out of bed took me at least a quarter of an hour."

Some equipment may be available to borrow. You may need to ask, and the earlier you do so, the more time the unit staff will have to find the equipment you need.

When can I eat?

After surgery postoperative patients are given fluids only to start with.

Although many hospitals do not give full meals after a caesarean, there is no reason for this restriction if a woman is recovering well and has no complications.

Hospitals generally cater for ill people and portions tend to be small – which can be a problem for new mothers. Ask for large helpings if you are hungry.

Make sure that your diet contains plenty of fibre and fluids, as constipation can be a problem. Encourage your visitors to bring fruit and other nourishing foods.

In some hospitals, you may be served meals in bed as a matter of course. In others, you may be expected to get up and go and eat in a dining area. If you find walking or sitting at a table difficult, you will need to discuss alternative arrangements.

If you cannot eat your meal when it arrives – perhaps because you are feeding your baby – ask if it can be kept warm or reheated later. There may be kitchen facilities available.

Remember to eat well if you are breastfeeding. You may want more food than you did when you were pregnant.

Will I have to use a bedpan?

Depending on hospital policy and your own circumstances, your catheter may be removed before

"Having not eaten since labour started on Saturday evening I was ravenous. i couldn't believe I wouldn't be given any food until the following day."

"I was busting, but just couldn't locate the right muscles. The midwife was great, we tried turning on taps, different positions, visualising waterfalls. The relief that came with success was blissful!"

you leave theatre but it is common to leave it in place for up to 24 hours. This is due to concerns about the return of bladder control and possible damage from excessive fluid retention, particularly if you have had a regional anaesthetic.

You may find it difficult to pass urine the first time after your operation, particularly if you are offered a bedpan. You may prefer to use a commode by the bedside or ask for help to the toilet.

Opening your bowels again for the first time can also be difficult. The timing varies considerably from woman to woman, and often does not happen for a week or more. Your midwives will ask you about this, and offer you a laxative or suppository if you have problems.

How soon can I get up?

One of the first challenges after a caesarean is standing. You should get plenty of assistance and encouragement from the midwives very soon after delivery and certainly within 24 hours. Moving around improves blood circulation and helps to prevent blood clots in your veins, which can cause serious problems such as deep vein thrombosis (DVT).

You will need to take your time, slowly moving your legs round, to reach a sitting position on the edge of your bed. If your bed is not low enough for your feet to reach the ground, ask your midwife to lower the bed or provide a step.

Standing upright can be unexpectedly difficult and feel almost impossible. You may have the characteristic 'caesarean stoop and shuffle'. It is usually better to stand as upright as possible.

"Nursing staff seemed totally preoccupied with ensuring I urinate, an exercise which involved struggling onto a commode, while in the most unbearable pain."

"It felt really sore pulling myself upright, but once there the position was better for back and morale than a stooped position. The hardest task was to get upright from lying, actually changing positions."

"I found that I could get out of bed easily but not get back in – it was discovered after three days the setting was too high for my height!"

Walking can be slow, exhausting and sometimes painful but gets easier the more often you try. It will also help you to recover quickly, both physically and emotionally.

Pain relief may mean you do not notice developing aches and pains, such as backache. You need to take extra care with your posture, especially when sitting or moving.

Try not to compare yourself with other women. If you had a difficult labour or other complications, your recovery may be slower.

If you usually have mobility difficulties or use a wheelchair, crutches or frame, discuss your needs with the staff. You will know what you need and what you feel able to do.

Can I have a bath?

Many women look forward to freshening up with a bath or shower after their baby is born. Although your operation is carried out under sterile conditions, you will be left with the remains of gel from the monitors and sticky patches from adhesive tape. You will also have bleeding, like a very heavy period (see *Will I bleed afterwards?* page 43).

At first, you are likely to be given a bed bath, until you are mobile enough to take a bath or shower. You may prefer to use a shower in hospital as there may be an increased risk of infection if you have a bath. Hospitals tend to develop strains of bacteria that are resistant to antibiotics. At home, having a bath does not carry the same risks as it does in hospital. You will tend to be immune to the bacteria in your own family home.

"With my husband to help, and by taking a plastic chair into the shower, I just about managed to wash properly before that scar started to burn too much."

If you are finding standing difficult, it may help to take a plastic chair into the shower, which you can sit or lean on. This also means you can wash your feet.

If you have been advised to keep support stockings on until you go home, it is usually all right to take them off while you have a shower. If you need help putting them back on again, ask your midwife.

You may also like to have a friend or partner to help you shower, even if only to reach the shampoo or towel. There should be a wheelchair-accessible shower for your use if needed.

What exercises should I do?

Many maternity units have an obstetric physiotherapist who offers specialist advice in postnatal exercise. Ideally, you should be able to see the physiotherapist and discuss your exercise needs personally. However, some units only provide exercise sheets.

At first, you may be recommended breathing exercises and ankle circling, both important after the operation.

Pelvic floor exercises are squeezing exercises that help to strengthen the pelvic floor muscles after birth. These exercises are important after both vaginal and caesarean birth to help prevent stress incontinence – the leaking of urine when you cough, laugh, sneeze or run.

Soon you will be able to start pelvic tilts lying on your back and then progress slowly to more strenuous exercise as your recovery allows.

"Before I was discharged the physiotherapist came round, shoved a leaflet in my hand about how to cope at home, getting out of chairs and your bed and walked off. I called her back and made her watch me – it turned out that some of my actions were wrong which would explain why I seemed to have a permanent stitch."

If you are unsure about a type of exercise, ask to see the obstetric physiotherapist, who will be happy to answer your questions. Specialist postnatal exercise classes suitable for all new mothers are available in some areas.

It's not advisable to start exercise routines that you did before you were pregnant until you have had your six-week postnatal examination, and many health professionals recommend waiting until 12 weeks after your baby is born.

Going home

How will I cope at home?

While some women appreciate the extra help available on the postnatal ward, many women look forward to the privacy and comfort of their own home. However, the return home can present additional challenges for caesarean mothers.

It will probably be the first time since your caesarean that you use stairs. You may find that you need to take these carefully and slowly, and plan what you carry up and down stairs – including your baby.

Some women have felt more secure sitting on the stairs and coming down on their bottom or coming down backwards. Others appreciate having their hands free to use the banister for support.

You may find that other simple tasks, such as refilling a kettle or getting up out of a chair, are also a strain. Heavier household tasks such as vacuuming, changing beds, ironing, or emptying the baby's bath are best avoided in the early weeks.

Tasks that involve stretching up, such as hanging laundry, reaching high cupboards or even changing a light bulb may also be beyond your capability for some time. If you have to bend down, for example to load the washing machine, it is better to bend your knees than bend your back.

Coping with a toddler or older child as well as a baby is likely to be very exhausting. You will need to take great care lifting or carrying the child. Think about a picnic on the floor rather than lifting your child into a high chair.

"I was so glad to get out of the hospital after four days and back home, even though I was nervous about being able to look after Josie."

"What surprised me most was the length of time it took to be completely pain free. Obviously the pain/discomfort lessened but even at six weeks I still took the odd paracetamol for pain when I had perhaps overdone it on a particular day."

It can often be helpful to have other people around – friends, family or someone else with a child of a similar age.

At home, you may find it useful to duplicate baby equipment. For example, you may find it easier to have nappy changing areas both upstairs and downstairs. Some women use their baby-changing bag at home as well as when out, and a raised surface such as a table is often helpful.

There are some adjustable baby change tables and cots available. Please contact Disability, Pregnancy and Parenting international (DPPi) for further information (see page 78).

Some women find it helpful to have a supply of drinks and snacks for themselves and their older children where they sit to feed their baby.

Baby seats or moses baskets may be difficult to move around, so you may want to have more than one, or make alternative sleeping arrangements for your baby. It is likely to be easier to take the baby out of the car seat, and move the baby and seat separately.

Many mothers find a baby carry sling makes carrying their baby easier.

You need to think about how you are going to bath your baby and whether you need anyone to help you. If you use a baby bath you are likely to need help to empty it. Some women wash their baby on their lap, so that they don't need to fill a bath.

Some parents choose to have their baby in the bath with them and like to have someone to help lift the baby in and out. Babies can also share baths with older siblings.

You will quickly find a method and ways of managing that work for you. Don't forget young babies and children don't need to be bathed every day!

What problems can occur during recovery?

Tell your midwife or family doctor as soon as possible if you suffer any undue pain or signs of possible infection, such as raised temperature, redness, soreness, discharge or a dragging sensation in your abdomen. This will help them rule out any rare but potentially serious complications.

Urine infections are more common after catheterisation and can usually be treated with a course of antibiotics.

Fungal infections, particularly thrush, can be a problem for some people after taking antibiotics. This can cause sore nipples and vaginal irritation. Treatments are available over the counter from pharmacists, or your GP will be able to diagnose and offer a longer course of treatment.

Although most women recover well from their caesarean, some find they are still experiencing pain or discomfort months (or in a few cases, years) later. Some women have found it difficult to get adequate medical help and they have had to be persistent.

When can I drive again?

After a caesarean, many women are advised not to drive for up to six weeks, although there are no clear restrictions. If you feel well enough, and you are capable of doing an emergency stop, check that your insurance will be valid. This may require medical clearance from your obstetrician or family doctor.

"The hospital acted very quickly and gave me antibiotics, but within a few weeks, I had thrush and a succession of even more ferocious urine infections."

"Because of the operation, when I came home I was very dependent on my family. I needed extra help with the chores and the baby as my movement and strength were severely restricted."

"It took four lots of antibiotics to finally clear my urinary tract infection, and this left me with thrush. No-one told me that this was common after a catheter!"

Not being able to drive can be one of the most frustrating limitations. You may also find it difficult to use public transport due to the walking and lifting that may be involved. Some mothers have found taking a taxi an easier solution.

Ask your health visitor or doctor's surgery if there are any local transport schemes.

Who can help?

After a caesarean you need extra support and help. Unfortunately, many people still misunderstand the needs of women who have had a caesarean operation.

Some people may treat you as helpless, while others expect you to be running around as if nothing has happened. Both extremes are usually unrealistic.

Each woman's individual needs are different and changeable. You may find it helpful to talk about your experience with friends, relatives, voluntary support groups and/or your health professionals.

Health professionals

If you have any questions about your operation, your labour, or your recovery, you should be able to go through your notes with one of the hospital midwives. You may also be able to talk with the midwife who cared for you.

You can consult your obstetrician if you have any serious post-caesarean complications or concerns. You can make an appointment yourself – you do not need a referral. Just phone the hospital and ask to speak to your obstetrician's secretary. Your obstetrician should also be able to give information about the operation and why it was necessary. If you feel it would be useful, you can ask to see the person who carried out your caesarean section.

Your community midwife will visit you until about ten days after the birth and may be able to continue to visit for up to 28 days, depending on how you are feeling and on your circumstances.

Your health visitor will usually take over from the midwife after about ten days. Health visitors will often visit you once or twice at home, so that you do not have to go out to the clinic in the early days.

Your family doctor is likely to carry out your six-week postnatal check, and be the person you consult if you have any medical concerns.

Your obstetric physiotherapist may be able to help if you are having difficulty with mobility.

Some units have clinical psychologists who are available to counsel women who have had difficult births.

If you have general questions about your health, NHS Direct (NHS 24 in Scotland) provides a 24–hour helpline service. The telephone numbers are on page 79.

Voluntary organisations

Voluntary organisations that may be able to help include local NCT branches, Good Neighbours schemes and community groups. Local services available may include:

- caesarean birth groups

- postnatal groups

- transport

- domestic help.

"NCT has been fantastic in their support after very traumatic emergency surgery. I would not be anywhere near so emotionally healthy without the support from the CS group or my local branch friends."

"I attended NCT antenatal classes and was well prepared for the number of people and what would be happening, I also had a lot of support from NCT members at coffee mornings."

Some of the National Childbirth Trust's 400 branches have caesarean birth groups or contacts. Those that don't should be able to find someone on their special experience register who has had a caesarean and who will be happy to talk to you.

What other practical help is available?

Think about things that will make your life easier and save you journeys, for example:

- shopping delivery
- nappy delivery
- cleaning and laundry services
- home hairdressing.

Most areas have good access to paid services that you can arrange on the phone or via the Internet.

Will the caesarean affect our sex life?

Sex can feel awkward for any couple after childbirth. The vaginal bleeding (see page 43) may persist for some weeks and you may both be tired, and find you have little time to yourselves.

You will often both be adjusting to new roles and sometimes birth experiences can affect relationships.

You may be in pain, or your partner may be afraid of hurting you. Fear of another pregnancy can also be a problem. Most couples find it helpful if they can discuss their feelings and worries about sex and their relationship.

How soon you have sex again after childbirth is a very personal decision and varies considerably between couples. Many couples do not go beyond cuddles and caresses for some time.

"I'm not too disappointed about having to have a caesarean. It was a very positive, happy experience. There were many benefits – no episiotomies or piles, no sitting on a rubber ring for days; a room to myself; and the resumption of a normal sex life after a couple of weeks."

If you have any concerns, you may want to talk to your family doctor or health visitor. If discomfort at the site of the scar continues beyond three to six months, then consider consulting an obstetrician.

If you wish to use an intrauterine device (IUD) or intrauterine system (IUS), you will need to find out how long it is advisable to wait before having one inserted. If you used a cap or diaphragm before you were pregnant, this will need refitting.

Sterilisation (tying or cutting the fallopian tubes) may be offered routinely to a woman having a third or subsequent caesarean. You should not feel under pressure to accept sterilisation. This cannot be done without your consent. When a man wants a vasectomy, he is usually advised to wait until his youngest child is at least six months old.

The NCT leaflet *Sex in pregnancy and after childbirth* (see page 75) discusses these issues in more depth.

Your emotions

Why did I have a caesarean?

A surprisingly large number of women leave hospital after a caesarean without understanding why they had the operation, and without having the chance to discuss what has happened.

You can make an appointment at any time postnatally with your obstetrician or midwife to discuss what happened and whether it is likely to affect future births.

You are legally entitled to a copy of your pregnancy labour and delivery notes, although you may be charged a fee for administrative costs. Please see the NCT information sheet *Records of your maternity care*, see page 75 for details.

How will I feel?

Every birth is different. Women experience birth in many ways, whether their baby is born vaginally or by caesarean section.

Experiences of caesarean birth vary, depending on the reasons for the caesarean and whether it was a planned or an emergency operation.

Your experience will be affected by whether you feel your questions have been answered and your wishes respected.

Many women are able to accept or feel very positively about a caesarean because they know it was the right option for them at the time and because they were fully involved in the decisions at all stages. Unfortunately, some women are left with nagging doubts about the reasons for their caesarean and whether it was really necessary.

"The first months of parenthood are so hectic that I hadn't really had time to think about what had happened. Now that it's all a year ago, I realise I still have a lot of questions about what happened and why I ended up having a caesarean."

Women have told us they found it helpful to:

- be able to talk about their operation
- know and understand the reasons for the operation
- have their experience valued by other people, such as carers and friends
- have had a spinal or epidural anaesthetic so that they were awake when their baby was born
- spend lots of time cuddling, looking at, talking to, and getting to know their baby
- keep some of the personal touches which may have been part of their original birth plan, including:
  - playing music
  - dimming the lights
  - being the first to discover the sex of the baby
  - being the first person to speak to their baby.

How will my partner feel?

Some partners find that a caesarean helps them feel involved and important. They may be the first to hold and greet the new baby, creating a strong and lasting bond.

Many fathers treasure feelings of awe, privilege, and closeness to the child that began with the first meeting.

In an emergency, staff may not have time to explain what is happening or to give support to the father, who may feel helpless or that he has failed in his role. Some partners may feel 'shut out' from their baby's birth.

"I had undergone surgery as one person and woken up as two – yet my brain and body hadn't registered this. The bonding was soon established once it had all 'connected'. But the feeling of having to complete labour remained with me for some time."

"For my husband, who had been with me all the time, it was not only a shock and a disappointment, but also extremely frightening. During this black hole in time, one of life's greatest experiences had taken place. Our daughter had been born, and neither I nor my husband had been there to experience it or greet her."

The depth of anxiety and loneliness that some men feel in this situation can be overpowering. A few men feel angry with the staff, or resentful towards the baby. If your partner feels upset, it may help him to talk to someone. You'll find information that may help in *What can I do to feel better?* on page 68.

When the caesarean is carried out under general anaesthetic, the father is often able to introduce the baby to the mother when she wakes up.

If the baby needs to go to special care, the father may be the best person to relay details of the baby's progress to the mother. However, he may also be asked to make decisions about the baby's care for which he feels ill prepared.

Some fathers say that their experience of the birth was not changed by the caesarean – they were by their partner's side, holding her hand, much as they had expected to be.

After the birth, they are more likely to be closely involved with caring for the baby so that the mother can recover. Changing nappies, bathing, dressing and soothing the baby can all help the father feel confident and really close to his baby.

Are negative feelings normal?

The range of feelings of caesarean mothers is very wide. Although some women feel very positive that their baby has been delivered safely, others can feel anything from mildly disappointed to severely traumatised.

Some women who experience negative feelings do so straight away, while others may not do so for months or even years.

"It feels a bit like I picked him up at the supermarket somehow – but I can't take him back and wouldn't want to!"

"I can't hide my feelings. I think it is essential for mothers like me to be 'allowed' to feel bad."

Feelings can include: guilt, anger, grief, or a sense of being cheated, betrayed, or abused.

The way you feel can be very much affected by the circumstances of the caesarean, and any labour. For example:

- Were you involved and comfortable with the decisions made?
- Do you think you had enough information?
- Were you treated with respect?

Many women find loss of control during birth very difficult to cope with. Women often wonder what they may have been able to do differently. 'What if...?' is a common question. Exploring such questions can help you come to terms with your experience and resolve your feelings.

It is normal to grieve for what you have lost. You are no longer pregnant, and if you were expecting – or hoping for – a normal birth you may feel robbed. Your body has changed. Many women feel a blow to their confidence and self-esteem.

If you feel control was taken away from you and you had things done to you against your wishes, or without your agreement, you may feel violated and bitterly hurt. You are not alone.

Different people cope in different ways:

- Some are able to acknowledge their feelings and move on, leaving the experience behind.
- Some are able to put the experience to one side until they are ready to revisit their feelings, while others are forced to do so by immediate demands, such as their baby being ill or the needs of older children.

"I lost a lot of friends, because I was so moody, temperamental, contradictory, had no sense of humour, could not let go of what had happened...I became a birth bore."

"I felt so vulnerable and hurt that I really did not want to see anyone, and if I had felt strong enough to take a stand, would not have seen anyone for at least a month. I released my residual anger and sent a withering letter to the obstetrician. I felt overwhelmed by the lack of understanding of what having a caesarean birth meant."

- Some need to deal with their feelings immediately – sometimes to the extent that it can be difficult to focus on anything else.

Will I get depressed?

Unless you feel very positively about your caesarean, you may find your emotions after caesarean birth confusing and overpowering, especially if you have had little time to prepare.

'Baby blues': It is common to experience 'baby blues' – a day or two when you feel weepy and upset for no obvious reason. This often happens about four or five days after the birth and can affect any new mother, whether her baby is born by caesarean or vaginally. Occasionally mothers take a few days or weeks to fall in love with their baby.

Postnatal depression affects 10–15% of all mothers.[18,19] It is more common after a traumatic birth. This condition is often linked to hormonal changes and can be treated. Your health visitor or GP will be able to help with a diagnosis.

Post Traumatic Stress Disorder (PTSD): Some women who have had a caesarean feel distressed about their experience and if the delivery was traumatic may suffer from PTSD (Post Traumatic Stress Disorder).

Although it was first recognised among soldiers and disaster victims, it has been shown that women can suffer PTSD following childbirth and gynaecological procedures.[20,21]

PTSD is not always recognised as such and may be confused with postnatal depression. PTSD is a response to events and is unlikely to be helped by drug treatment.

"I was fine so how could I complain? This was clearly the view of the medical staff and showed in their comments and behaviour towards me. Their reaction to my distress exacerbated it."

"I lived in two worlds, the 'videotape' of the birth and the 'real' world. The videotape felt more real. I lived in an air bubble, not quite connecting with anyone. I could hear and communicate, but I experienced interaction with others as a spectator."

Unfortunately, PTSD is rarely diagnosed and the symptoms may overlap with those of depression. Symptoms of PTSD include:

- disturbing memories of the birth experience
- flashbacks (sudden and vivid memories)
- nightmares
- sadness
- fearfulness
- anxiety
- irritability
- feeling numb
- feeling detached
- obsessive thoughts about the birth
- amnesia (inability to recall important aspects of the birth event)
- jumpiness and being easily startled
- avoiding all reminders of the birth
- intense psychological stress at exposure to events that resemble the birth
- significant difficulties in resuming sex
- hypersensitivity to injustice.

Unfortunately, PTSD is not widely known, recognised or understood, and some mothers struggle to find anyone who understands (see *Further support and information*, pages 75-79).

"I wanted to help everyone and prevent them from having to go through what I had just been through."

"I became super sensitive, from the slightest criticism, to a shade or smell that reminded me of the hospital, and I was sent back to the horror."

"Nightmares would engulf me. I would wake up to find my pillow soaked and tears still rolling down my face."

What can I do to feel better?

Recovery from traumatic or difficult experiences usually involves completing your understanding of events. Some women need to go over every detail, while others only want a broad understanding.

You may need to go over the facts of what happened and to understand the words and actions of others at the time. With this comes the realisation that your reactions and feelings are normal and reasonable.

Two elements play an important part in recovery from a difficult or traumatic birth experience:

- information to help you piece together what happened and why

- being listened to and supported by somebody who understands.

Information

You can ask to go through your notes with a midwife. Some hospitals offer this service under names such as 'Birth Afterthoughts' or 'Birth Reflections'. You should still be able to discuss your birth and your care, even if your hospital does not offer it as a named service.

If you have a complaint or nagging doubts about your care, you can call the unit where you had your baby and ask for an appointment to see the supervisor of midwives or another senior midwife. They should be sympathetic and able to respond to your concerns.

If an NHS midwife does not seem to be able to help you, you could consider discussing your care with a private, independent midwife (see page 78 for

"When I saw a psychiatrist, I was so scared about him thinking that I was a lunatic, I did my best to be 'normal' and to play down my symptoms and the severity of them. Fortunately he saw through me and I finally had acknowledgement that I really was not mad."

"When the babies were nine months old I contacted a counsellor; she recognised my symptoms as those caused by trauma. This was an enormous relief, at least I wasn't going mad."

details). You are legally entitled to a copy of your pregnancy, labour and delivery notes. NCT and AIMS produce details of how to access your notes. Their addresses are on pages 75 and 76.

You can make an appointment with your obstetrician to discuss your case – you do not need a referral.

You can research aspects of what happened from printed material or via the Internet. See pages 75-83 for a suggested reading list and websites.

Support

Being listened to by somebody who understands can be very important. Often family and friends will not understand your need to go over and over an event which you obviously find distressing. They may think you should move on. People who will listen to you include:

- a psychotherapist or counsellor, arranged either privately or via your GP. Psychotherapists explore issues in depth. Counselling can be very helpful, or it can be disappointing if the counsellor does not sufficiently understand birth issues. To find a psychotherapist in your area, see page 77 for details.

- support organisations such as the NCT, AIMS, or the Birth Crisis Network. These organisations offer the opportunity to talk through what happened with someone who understands and who may have helpful information.

- other women who feel the same way, either face-to-face in local mother and baby groups or in online discussion groups. See page 77 for details.

"I found support in the most surprising place – at our local homebirth support group meeting; they understood what I had missed."

Coming to terms with a difficult experience is a personal journey. On the positive side, you are in control, and can choose your direction and speed, and who you wish to seek help from.

It is likely that you will need a variety of sources of information and support. Please see pages 75-83.

The future

Might this caesarean affect future births?

Although most caesarean decisions are based on circumstances surrounding the current birth, future births may be affected.

Caesarean delivery can affect fertility. Women who have had a caesarean birth are known to have fewer children, though the reasons for this are not clear. They also take longer to conceive again.[22,23]

Complications affecting the placenta, although uncommon, are more frequent after a caesarean. Rates of placental problems also increase with the number of previous caesareans, but again, the rate remains very small.

If the caesarean was your first birth, any subsequent labour will effectively be a first time labour from the point that you reached before the caesarean. Health professionals and parents often forget this.

When the uterus carries a scar there is a small risk of separation, which increases the risk of uterine rupture in another pregnancy. For this reason, health professionals often impose conditions on subsequent labours. However, the care of a women in labour after a previous lower-segment caesarean section should be little different from that of any woman in labour.[24]

Can I have my next baby normally?

Vaginal birth after caesarean is generally referred to as VBAC (pronounced 'veeback'). Some health professionals call it 'trial of labour' or 'trial of scar'.

Placenta praevia: when the placenta lies across, or less than two centimetres from the neck of the uterus towards the end of pregnancy or when labour starts.

Placenta accreta: where the placenta is abnormally stuck to the uterus, usually requiring manual removal bit by bit and causing haemorrhage (bleeding). A hysterectomy may be necessary.

There are very few reasons why a repeat caesarean might be necessary. If there is no medical reason not to have a vaginal birth, VBAC is a safe option for your baby.

Women whose first babies were born by caesarean when the pelvis was suspected to be too small have gone on to give birth vaginally to larger babies.

The likelihood of women successfully having a vaginal birth after more than one previous caesarean is about the same as that for women who have had only one previous section. Unfortunately, many health professionals still expect such women to have a repeat caesarean with subsequent babies.

The main concern about VBAC is that the scar could separate and lead to a uterine rupture. Some scar separation can happen without causing any labour or birth problem. However, a uterine rupture is serious and can put the life of mother and baby at risk. Uterine rupture occurs in about 1 in 200 VBAC labours. A caesarean will be carried out and the uterus can usually be repaired.

How many caesareans can I have?

Women who would like a large family are often worried that birth by caesarean may limit the number of children they can have.

There is no absolute limit to the number of caesareans that can be performed, although the more caesareans a woman has had, the more scar tissue may have built up, making further operations more difficult to perform. However, everyone heals differently. If you are worried, it may help to discuss this with your obstetrician.

Women who have had three, four or more caesareans will almost certainly be offered a section for another birth.

There is also a very small increased risk of placental problems the more caesareans a woman has. These include placenta praevia and placenta accreta, when the placenta is badly positioned or has grown into the wall of the uterus.

How soon can I get pregnant again?

Many women worry that if they get pregnant again soon after a caesarean that the scar will not be strong enough.

Although, according to one source, the wound in your uterus will heal almost fully by about six weeks, more recent evidence shows that the uterine scar seems to become stronger over time. Small reductions in scar rupture rates are seen as the time between pregnancies increases from 6 to 24 months.[25,26]

However, the risks are small in all cases and the length of time after a caesarean that you become pregnant should not make a significant difference to the pregnancy or birth.

It is also important to consider how physically and emotionally recovered you feel to cope with another pregnancy. It is a very personal decision.

A short gap between pregnancies should not rule out a vaginal birth. Many women have had a second baby vaginally within a year of their caesarean. There is a lot of information available on VBAC and it is very encouraging. To find out more, see the NCT information sheet *Vaginal birth after caesarean* and the list of support organisations on pages 75-79.

"I have had four elective caesareans, and I can only say they are getting better."

"I had been told another caesarean would be necessary, but when I discussed this further, it was agreed I could have a 'trial of labour'. It all went so well, and I'm glad I questioned things."

References

1. National Collaborating Centre for Women's and Children's Health, commissioned by the National Institute for Clinical Excellence (NICE). *Caesarean Section Clinical Guideline* London, RCOG Press; 2004.

2. Thomas J, Paranjothy S, Royal College of Obstetricians and Gynaecologists Clinical Effectiveness Support Unit. *National sentinel caesarean section audit report.* London: RCOG Press; 2001.

3. Hannah ME, Hannah WJ, Hewson SA, et al. Planned caesarean section versus planned vaginal birth for breech presentation at term: a randomised multicentre trial. Term Breech Trial Collaborative Group. *Lancet* 2000;356(9239):1375-83.

4. Hofmeyr GJ, Hannah ME. Planned caesarean section for term breech delivery (Cochrane Review). In: *The Cochrane Library*, Issue 2, 2004. Available on www.nelh.nhs.uk/cochrane

5. Keirse, MJ. Evidence-based childbirth only for breech babies? *Birth* 2002 Mar;29(1):55-9.

6. Simkin PT. Maternal positions and pelves revisited. *Birth* 2003 June; 30(2) 130-2. Critique of Michel SC, Rake A, Treiber K, et al. MR obstetric pelvimetry: Effect of birthing position on pelvic bony dimensions. *Am J Roentgenol* 2002 Oct;179(4):1063-7.

7. Albers LL. Monitoring the fetus in labor: evidence to support the methods. *J Midwifery Womens Health* 2001;46(6):366-73.

8. Royal College of Obstetricians and Gynaecologists/Clinical Effectiveness Support Unit. Evidence-Based Clinical Guideline no 8. The use of electronic fetal monitoring. Updated May 2001. Available on: www.rcog.org.uk/resources/pdf/efm_guideline_final_2may2001.pdf

9. Royal College of Obstetricians and Gynaecologists. Green Top Clinical Guideline no 30. Management of genital herpes in pregnancy. Updated March 2002. Available on: www.rcog.org.uk/resources/Public/Genital_Herpes_No30.pdf

10. Brocklehurst P. Interventions for reducing the risk of mother-to-child transmission of HIV infection. (Cochrane Review). In: *The Cochrane Library*, Issue 3, 2003. Oxford: Update Software. Available on: www.nelh.nhs.uk/cochrane

11. O'Brien-Abel N. Uterine rupture during VBAC trial of labor: risk factors and fetal response. *J Midwifery Womens Health* 2003;48(4):249-57.

12. Roberts LJ. Elective section after two sections – where's the evidence? *Br J Obstet Gynaecol* 1991;98(12):1199-202.

13. Lewis G, Drife J. *Why do mothers die?* 1997-1999: The fifth report of the Confidential Enquiries into Maternal Deaths in the United Kingdom. London: RCOG Press; 2001.

14. Lee S, Hassan A, Ingram D et al. Effects of different modes of delivery on lung volumes of newborn infants. *Pediatr Pulmonol* 1999;27(5):318-21.

15. Patel H, Beeby PJ, Henderson-Smart DJ. Predicting the need for ventilatory support in neonates 30–36 weeks' gestational age. *J Paediatr Child Health* 2003;39(3):206-9.

16. Morrison JJ, Rennie JM, Milton PJ. Neonatal respiratory morbidity and mode of delivery at term: influence of timing of elective caesarean section. *Br J Obstet Gynaecol* 1995;102(2):101-6.

17. Smaill F, Hofmeyr GJ. Antibiotic prophylaxis for cesarean section (Cochrane Review). In: *The Cochrane Library*, Issue 3, 2003. Oxford: Update Software. Available on www.nelh.nhs.uk/cochrane

18. Royal College of Obstetricians and Gynaecologists, Royal College of Midwives, and National Childbirth Trust. The rising caesarean rate - causes and effects for public health. Report of a national conference organised by the RCOG; RCM; NCT held in London on 7 November 2000. London: National Childbirth Trust; 2001.

19. Scottish Intercollegiate Guidelines Network. No 60 2002. *Postnatal depression and puerperal psychosis:* a national clinical guideline. www.sign.ac.uk/guidelines/fulltext/60/index.html

20. Menage J. Post-traumatic stress disorder in women who have undergone obstetric and/or gynaecological procedures. *J Reprod Infant Psych* 1993;11:221-8.

21. Ballard CG, Stanley AK, Brockington IF. Post-traumatic stress disorder (PTSD) after childbirth. *Br J Psychia* 1995;166:525-8.

22. Murphy DJ, Stirrat GM, Heron J et al. The relationship between caesarean section and subfertility in a population-based sample of 14,541 pregnancies. *Hum Reprod* 2002;17(4):1914-7.

23. Bahl R, Strachan B, Murphy DJ. Outcome of subsequent pregnancy three years after previous operative delivery in the second stage of labour: cohort study. *BMJ* 2004;328(7435):311.

24. Enkin M, Keirse MJ, Neilson J et al. A Guide to Effective Care in Pregnancy and Childbirth. Oxford: Oxford University Press; 2000.

25. Shipp TD, Zelop CM, Repke JT et al. Interdelivery interval and risk of symptomatic uterine rupture. *Obstet Gynecol* 2001;97(2):175-7.

26. Bujold E, Mehta SH, Bujold C et al. Interdelivery interval and uterine rupture. *Am J Obstet Gynecol* 2002;187(5):1199-202.

Further support and information

National Childbirth Trust (NCT)

Alexandra House
Oldham Terrace
London W3 6NH

Enquiry line: 0870 444 8707
(Mon-Thu 9am-5pm, Fri 9am- 4pm)

Breastfeeding line: 0870 444 8708
(7 days 8am-10pm)

www.nctpregnancyandbabycare.com

E-mail: enquiries@national-childbirth-trust.co.uk

If your questions about caesarean birth have not been answered in this booklet, NCT's National Caesarean Birth and VBAC Co-ordinators can offer further help. You can reach them by contacting the NCT by phone, e-mail or the website.

Some of our local NCT branches have caesarean birth groups or caesarean birth contacts. Those that do not may be able to find someone on their special experience register who will be happy to talk.

Some branches also have antenatal teachers who will be able to discuss caesarean matters with you, both before and after the birth.

NCT Sales Ltd

239 Shawbridge Street
Glasgow G43 1QN

Phone: 0870 112 1120

www.nctms.co.uk

E-mail: sales@nctms.co.uk

Fax: 0141 636 0606

NCT information sheets relevant to this booklet include:

- Breech baby
- Records of your maternity care
- Sex in pregnancy and after childbirth
- Vaginal birth after caesarean
- Breastfeeding - how to express and store your milk
- Breastfeeding - a good start
- Straightforward birth.

These and all other NCT publications are available from NCT Sales, who also have details of the comfortable knickers and nightwear mentioned on page 49.

Action on Pre-Eclampsia (APEC)

84-88 Pinner Road
Harrow
Middlesex HA1 4HZ

Helpline: 020 8427 4217

www.apec.org.uk

E-mail: enquiries@apec.org.uk

Fax: 020 8424 0653

Raises awareness about pre-eclampsia among parents and health professionals; supports sufferers; promotes medical research into the disease.

Active Birth Centre

25 Bickerton Road
London N19 5JT

Phone: 020 7281 6760
(Mon-Fri, 9am-5pm)

www.activebirthcentre.com

E-mail: mail@activebirthcentre.com

Fax: 020 7263 8098

Helps parents-to-be to explore alternatives and increase self-awareness and understanding in order to have the best possible experience of pregnancy, labour and birth.

Association for Improvements in Maternity Services (AIMS)

5 Ann's Court
Grove Road
Surbiton
Surrey KT6 4BE

Helpline: 0870 765 1433

Fax: 0870 765 1454

www.aims.org.uk

Supports parents and professionals in the UK and Ireland.

Association for Postnatal Illness (APNI)

145 Dawes Road
London SW6 7EB

Phone: 020 7386 0868 (Mon and Fri 10am-2pm,Tue, Wed, Thur 10am-5pm)

www.apni.org

E-mail: info@apni.org

Fax: 020 7386 8885

Advises and supports women suffering from postnatal depression.

Association of Breastfeeding Mothers

PO Box 207
Bridgwater
Somerset TA6 7YT

Helpline 020 7813 1481

www.abm.me.uk

E-mail: info@abm.me.uk

Run by mothers for mothers, committed to giving friendly support and supplying accurate information to all women wishing to breastfeed.

Birth Choice UK

www.birthchoiceuk.com

Helps women choose where to have their baby. Gives information on maternity care options, your local hospital's 'normal birth' rate, official NHS maternity statistics and summaries of evidence-based research.

Birth Crisis Network

Phone: 01865 300 266

(answerphone: calls will be responded to within 24 hours)

www.sheilakitzinger.com/Birth%20Crisis.htm

Offers reflective listening to women who want to talk about a traumatic birth.

Birthrites: Healing After a Caesarean

www.birthrites.edsite.com.au

An Australian website on various aspects of caesarean birth and VBAC.

BLISS – the premature baby charity

68 South Lambeth Road
London SW8 1RL

Phone: (for general calls from both parents and health professionals) 0870 770 0337 (Mon-Fri, 9am-5.30pm)

Freephone helpline: (for anxious or distressed parents) 0500 618140 (Mon-Fri, 10am-5pm, but callers can leave a message at other times)

www.bliss.org.uk

E-mail: information@bliss.org.uk

Fax: 0870 7700 338

Supports parents of babies in special and intensive care.

The Breastfeeding Network (BfN)

PO Box 11126
Paisley PA2 8YB

SupporterLine: 0870 900 8787

www.breastfeedingnetwork.org.uk

E-Mail: email@breastfeedingnetwork.org.uk

Support and information for breastfeeding women.

British Association of Psychotherapists

37 Mapesbury Road
London NW2 4HJ

Phone: 020 8452 9823

Fax: 020 8452 0310

www.bap-psychotherapy.org/

E-mail: mail@bap-psychotherapy.org

May help to locate a psychotherapist if you want to talk to a professional in depth about your birth experience.

Caesarean and VBAC Information

www.caesarean.org.uk

E-mail: gina@caesarean.org.uk or debbie@caesarean.org.uk

Information and articles relating to all aspects of caesarean and VBAC birth, including caesarean scar pictures. (Site owned by two of the authors of this book).

Caesarean E-groups

There are several e-groups for those interested in caesarean birth or VBAC. They include:

http://groups.yahoo.com/group/nct-caesarean-planning

http://groups.yahoo.com/group/nct-caesarean

E-groups provide e-mail contact with the group as all members receive all e-mails posted to the group. Joining involves a simple registration process.

Caesarean Support Network

55 Cooil Drive
Douglas
Isle of Man IM2 2HF

Phone: 01624 661 269 (evenings and weekends)

E-mail: yvonnewilliams@manx.net

Listens to, helps and offers support to women who have had or may need to have a caesarean section.

Disability, Pregnancy and Parenthood international (DPPi)

Unit F9, 89-93 Fonthill Road
London N4 3JH

Phone: 0800 018 4730

www.dppi.org.uk

E-mail: info@dppi.org.uk

Fax: 020 7263 6399

Practical information, for example on bathing or lifting your baby. At the same address and telephone number is the National Centre for Disabled Parents. This organisation gives one-to-one support with ongoing issues such as assessments or complaints.

Disabled Parents Network

Unit F9, 89-93 Fonthill Road
London N4 3JH

Phone: 0870 241 0450

Text: 0800 018 9949

Fax: 020 7263 6399

www.disabledparentsnetwork.org.uk/

E-mail:information@disabledparents network.org.uk

Disabled parent-to-disabled parent support.

Doula UK

PO Box 26678
London N14 4WB

www.doula.org.uk

E-mail: info@doula.org.uk

Provides emotional and practical support to enable a woman to have the most satisfying time that she can during pregnancy, birth and the early days as a new mum.

Fathers Direct

Herald House, Lambs Passage, Bunhill Row
London EC1Y 8TQ

Phone: 020 7920 9491

Fax: 020 7374 2966

www.fathersdirect.com

E-mail: enquiries@fathersdirect.com

UK national information centre for fatherhood. Website has booklists, useful links, forums and information for new fathers.

Homebirth Reference Site

www.homebirth.org.uk

angela@homebirth.org.uk

Provides information about homebirth, including birth stories and how to book a homebirth in the UK. Also includes statistical information on VBAC.

Independent Midwives Association

1 The Great Quarry
Guildford
Surrey GU1 3XN

Phone: 01483 821 104

information@independentmidwives.org.uk

E-mail: c.f.winter@bournemouth.ac.uk

Has a register of independent midwives in England, Wales and Scotland.

La Leche League (Great Britain)

PO Box 29
West Bridgford
Nottingham
NG2 7NP

Phone: 0845 120 2918

www.laleche.org.uk

E-mail:lllgb@wsds.co.uk

Helps mothers to breastfeed through mother-to-mother support, encouragement, information and education.

NHS Direct

England: Phone: 0845 4647

www.nhsdirect.nhs.uk/

Wales: Phone: 0845 4647

www.nhsdirect.wales.nhs.uk/

NHS 24 (Scotland)

Phone: 0845 4242424

Teams of nurse advisors give telephone advice. The NHS Direct website asks you about symptoms step-by-step and suggests action you may take.

Pre-Eclampsia Society

Rhianfa

Carmel

Caernarfon

Gwynedd LL54 7RL

Phone: 01286 882685

www.dawnjames.clara.net

E-mail: dawnjames@clara.co.uk

Support network.

REMAP

Hazeldene

Ightham

Sevenoaks

Kent TN15 9AD

Phone: 0845 130 0456

Fax: 0845 130 0789

www.remap.org.uk

E-mail: info@remap.org.uk

Supplies equipment (including adjustable baby cribs) for disabled parents.

REMAP (Scotland)

Maulside Lodge

Beith

Ayrshire KA15 1JJ

Phone: 01294 832566

Fax: 01294 834162

Supplies equipment (including adjustable baby cribs) for disabled parents in Scotland.

Royal College of Anaesthetists

Publish a number of leaflets about spinal, general and epidural anaesthetics. These are available to download on

www.youranaesthetic.info

Stillbirth and Neonatal Death Society (SANDS)

28 Portland Place

London W1B 1LY

Helpline: 020 7436 5881 (Mon-Fri, 10am-3pm)

www.uk-sands.org

E-mail: support@uk-sands.org

Support for bereaved parents and their families when their baby dies at or soon after birth.

Twins and Multiple Births Association (TAMBA)

2 The Willows

Gardner Road

Guildford

Surrey GU1 4PG

Phone: 0870 770 3305

Mon-Fri, 9.30am-5pm

www.tamba.org.uk

E-mail: enquiries@tamba.org.uk

Aims to provide information and mutual support networks for families of twins, triplets and more, highlighting their unique needs to all involved in their care.

VBAC Pages (on the UK homebirth reference suite website)

www.vbac.org.uk

Provides information about VBAC, including statistics and birth stories.

Further reading

Some books may be difficult to obtain or out of print; however it is possible to borrow any book from your public library. If a particular book is not available locally, it can be requested for you. Some NCT branches and NCT antenatal teachers may have copies they can lend.

Caesarean birth

The Caesarean Experience

Sarah Clement

London: Pandora: 1995. ISBN: 0044407386

Sarah is a psychologist and caesarean mother. Covers all aspects of caesarean birth, including the emotional effects.

Caesarean Recovery

Chrissie Gallagher-Mundy

London: Carroll & Brown, 2004.

ISBN 1903258723

Day-by-day guide to exercising after a caesarean section, beautifully illustrated.

Vaginal birth after caesarean section (VBAC)

Birth after Caesarean

Jenny Lesley

London: AIMS, 2004. ISBN 1874413177

Provides information about choices, suggests ways in which VBAC can be made more likely and informs women about their rights and where to find support.

Natural Childbirth After Cesarean

Karis Crawford and Johanne Walters

Cambridge, MA: Blackwell Science: 1996.
ISBN: 086542490X

In this American book, which gives good guidance on preparation for VBAC, 'natural' means vaginal.

The VBAC Companion:The expectant mother's guide to vaginal birth after cesarean

Diana Korte

Boston, MA: Harvard Common Press; 1998. ISBN: 1558321292

An American book which explains the risks and benefits of both repeat caesareans and vaginal births after a caesarean, including overcoming fears.

Vaginal Birth After Cesarean:The smart woman's guide to vaginal birth after cesarean

Elizabeth Kaufmann

Alameda, CA: Hunter House; 1996.
ISBN: 0897932021

Provides guidance for women wondering about giving birth naturally after having a caesarean section, from coping with the inevitable negative opinions about VBAC to choosing the right caregiver.

The Vaginal Birth After Cesarean (VBAC) Experience: Birth stories by parents and professionals

Lynn Baptisti Richards

Westport, CT: Bergin & Garvey; 1987.
ISBN: 0897891201

Shares the observations of mothers, doctors and midwives on vaginal and cesarean births and offers a critical look at birthing practices in the USA.

Trust your body! Trust your baby!

Childbirth wisdom and cesarean prevention

Andrea Frank Henkart

Westport, CT: Greenwood Press; 1995.
ISBN: 0897892941

Henkart and her collaborators look at how the system causes caesareans and how they might be avoided. Another book from the USA.

Silent Knife: cesarean prevention and vaginal birth after cesarean (VBAC).

Nancy Wainer Cohen, Lois J Estner

South Hadley, MA: Bergin & Garvey; 1983.
ISBN:0897890272

This classic American book is still relevant today, much of the research base has not been superseded. May seem rather aggressive, but very to the point.

Anaesthesia and pain relief

Pain relief in labour

Caesarean section – your choice of anaesthesia

Obstetric Anaesthetists' Association

Ask your obstetrician for a copy, or download from www.oaa-anaes.ac.uk

General birth

Birth Words: some pregnancy and childbirth words and what they mean

National Childbirth Trust.

London: The National Childbirth Trust; 1995. ISBN: 1870129679

An illustrated booklet offering simple definitions of pregnancy and childbirth terms.

Early Days: life with a new baby

National Childbirth Trust.

London, National Childbirth Trust. 2003.

Covers getting organised, coping with tiredness, basics of baby care - and talks about your body, your feelings and your relationships.

Feelings After Birth: the NCT book of postnatal depression

Heather Welford
London: NCT Publishing; 2002.
ISBN: 0954301803

Sex in Pregnancy and After Childbirth

National Childbirth Trust.

London, National Childbirth Trust. 1996.
ISBN: 1870129695

Safer Childbirth?

A critical history of maternity care

Marjorie Tew

3rd edition. London: Free Association Books Ltd; 1998.
ISBN: 1853434264

This third edition considers the evidence on which the author's recommended changes in policy were made and the implications of implementing them. Statistics suggested that for some women hospital birth might actually be more dangerous than home birth.

What's right for me? Making decisions in pregnancy and birth

Sara Wickham

London: AIMS; 2002. ISBN: 1874413134

This publication from the Association for Improvements in the Maternity Services is different from other books on women's choices during pregnancy. It outlines the principles of making birth choices, rather than focusing on giving alternative options to maternity care. It raises many issues that women might want to consider when thinking about the decisions they have to make, including informed choice, coercion, and sources of information.

Maternal and Parental Rights

Katie Wood

Legal Guidance Series. London: The Stationery Office Books; 2001. ISBN: 0117025526

Birth Your Way: Choosing birth at home or in a birth centre

Sheila Kitzinger

London: Dorling Kindersley; 2002.
ISBN: 0751307882

As research discloses the risks of intensively managed hospital births, increasing numbers of women are considering alternatives. This updated guide includes first-hand accounts of women's experiences of birth, and should help those who want to make the right decision confidently for themselves.

Birthing From Within

Pam England and Rob Horowitz

Albuquerque, NM: Partera Press; 1998.
ISBN: 0965987302

An approach to birth that seeks to prepare a mother for birthing from within. Everything is covered, from caesarean deliveries to pain medications and endorphins. This book offers insight into what a mother will need to know about labour and birth from her perspective.

Evidence-based practice

NICE Caesarean Guidline

National Collaborating Centre for Women's and Children's Health, commissioned by the National Institute for Clinical Excellence (NICE). London, RCOG Press; 2004.

ISBN: 1904752020

These clinical guidelines are available in several forms. Healthcare professionals should be using the guideline and providing evidence-based information and care options as recommended in it.

Caesarean section: Understanding NICE guidance

This booklet summarises the information in the NICE guidelines for pregnant women, their partners and the public.

You can order a copy of the booklet from the NHS Response Line, 0870 1555 455 and quote reference number N0479 (N0480 for a version in Welsh and English).

For a full list of publications for health professionals and the public, visit www.nice.org.uk

The Cochrane Library

The Cochrane Library consists of a regularly updated collection of evidence-based information, including reviews on topics such as breech presentation, antibiotic use, twin deliveries, caesarean techniques and eating and drinking after a caesarean.

www.nelh.nhs.uk.cochrane.asp

Guide to Effective Care in Pregnancy and Childbirth

Murray Enkin and others

3rd edition. New York: Oxford University Press; 2000. ISBN: 019263173X

This guide provides a highly reliable guide to research evidence on the effects of the various care practices carried out during pregnancy, childbirth and the early days after birth.

MIDIRS Informed Choice

MIDIRS produce various leaflets on pregnancy and birth topics, including breech presentation and going overdue.

www.midirs.org/nelh/nelh.nsf/icnview2c

Statistics and trends in caesarean birth

National Sentinel Caesarean Section Audit Report

Thomas J, Paranjothy S, Royal College of Obstetricians and Gynaecologists Clinical Effectiveness Support Unit. London: RCOG Press; 2001. ISBN: 1900364662 www.rcog.org.uk/mainpages.asp?PageID=114

Statistical analysis of all caesareans carried out in a three-month period in England, Wales, Northern Ireland, Channel Islands and the Isle of Man.

Expert Advisory Group on Caesarean Section in Scotland 2001.
www.show.scot.nhs.uk/crag/topics/reprod/ EAG1.htm

A review of the recent trend of caesarean section in Scotland.

The rising caesarean rate

- A public health issue
- Causes and effects for public health
- From audit to action

Three reports of national conferences organised by the National Childbirth Trust, the Royal College of Midwives and the Royal College of Obstetricians and Gynaecologists.